© Copyright 2021 -All rights reserved.

The content contained within this book may not be reproduced, duplicated or transmitted without direct written permission from the author or the publisher.

Under no circumstances will any blame or legal responsibility be held against the publisher, or author, for any damages, reparation, or monetary loss due to the information contained within this book, either directly or indirectly.

Legal Notice:

This book is copyright protected. It is only for personal use. You cannot amend, distribute, sell, use, quote or paraphrase any part, or the content within this book, without the consent of the author or publisher.

Disclaimer Notice:

Please note the information contained within this document is for educational and entertainment purposes only. All effort has been executed to present accurate, up to date, reliable, complete information. No warranties of any kind are declared or implied. Readers acknowledge that the author is not engaged in the rendering of legal, financial, medical or professional advice. The content within this book has been derived from various sources. Please consult a licensed professional before attempting any techniques outlined in this book.

By reading this document, the reader agrees that under no circumstances is the author responsible for any losses, direct or indirect, that are incurred as a result of the use of the information contained within this document, including, but not limited to, errors, omissions, or inaccuracies.

TABLE OF CONTENTS

INTRODUCTION 4

CHAPTER 1: 6
RESISTANCE BANDS
Power Resistance Loop
Bands 6
Mini Loop Bands 6
Tube Bands 7
Therapy Bands 7
Resistance Band Levels 7

CHAPTER 2: 8
GAUGING YOUR LEVEL
Beginner 8
Intermediate 9
Advanced 9

CHAPTER 3: 10
BEFORE YOU BEGIN
Stretching and Warming Up .. 10
Breathing 10
Quality Over Quantity 10
Progressive Overload 11
Basic Gym Terms 11

CHAPTER 4: 12
HOW TO USE THIS BOOK
Basic 5 Minute Warm-Up
Routine 13

CHAPTER 5: 14
CHEST
Resistance Band Push-Ups 14
Standing Lower Chest Fly 15
Resistance Band Chest
Press 16
Lying Chest Press 17
Lying Wide Chest Press 18
Lying Crush Press 19
Resistance Band Pullover 20
Kneeling Band Chest Flys 21
Valley Press 22
Standing Incline Wide Fly 23
Alternate Chest Punches 24

CHAPTER 6: 25
SHOULDERS
Reverse Flys 25
Face Pulls 26
Overhead Raise 27
Frontal Raise 28

Resistance Band Shoulder
Press 29
Lateral Raise 30
Resistance Band Stretches 31
Internal Pull-ins 32
External Pull-ins 33
Pull Downs 34
Rectangular Raises 35
One Arm Skis 36

CHAPTER 7: 37
BACK
Resistance Band Row 37
Banded Bent-over Rows 38
Banded Bent-Over Under-
Hand Rows 39
Elevated Under-Hand Rows .. 40
Elevated Rows 41
Rear Delt Pull-Outs 42
Elevated Straight Arm
Pulldowns 43
Elevated Side-Arm
Pulldowns 44
Banded Romanian Deadlift .. 45
Single-Arm Rows 46
Bent-Over Back Flys 47
Seated Pronated Rows 48
Seated Reverse Rows 49
Banded Trap Shrugs 50

CHAPTER 8: 51
ARMS
Banded Push Downs-
Triceps 51
Banded Tricep Extensions-
Triceps 52
Banded Pullbacks-Triceps 53
Side Single-Arm Extensions-
Triceps 54
Mini Banded Pull Downs-
Triceps 55
Banded Close Grip Push-Ups-
Triceps 56
Banded Curls-Biceps 57
Kneeling Single-Arm Curls-
Biceps 58
Banded Wide Curls-Biceps ... 59
Banded Alternating Curls With
Static Hold-Biceps 60

Bent-over Banded Curls-
Biceps 61
Banded Hammer Curls-
Biceps 62
Seated Banded Wrist Curls-
Forearms 63
Seated Banded Pronated Wrist
Curls-Forearms 64
Standing Banded Wrist Curls-
Forearms 65
Standing Banded Pronated
Wrist Curls-Forearms 66
Standing Wrist Circles-
Forearms 67

CHAPTER 9: 68
LEGS
Banded Glute Bridges 68
Banded Squats 69
Squat and Jump 70
Lateral Side Steps 71
Banded Kickbacks 72
Banded Side Leg Lifts 73
Mid-bridge In & Outs 74
Banded Back Lunges 75
Tabletop Side Leg Raises 76
Banded Tabletop Kickbacks .. 77
Banded Calf Raises 78
Banded Squat Calf Raises 79

CHAPTER 10: 80
CORE
Banded Russian Twists 80
Banded Lying Leg Raises 81
Banded Lying Knee
Tuck Ins 82
Banded Bicycles 83
Banded Scissor Kicks 84
Banded Side Plank Raises 85
Standing Oblique Twists 86
Kneeling Angled Oblique
Twists 87
Banded Lying Toe Touches .. 88
Banded Flutter Kicks 89
Banded Boat Hold 90

ALL IN ALL... 91
REFERENCES 92

INTRODUCTION

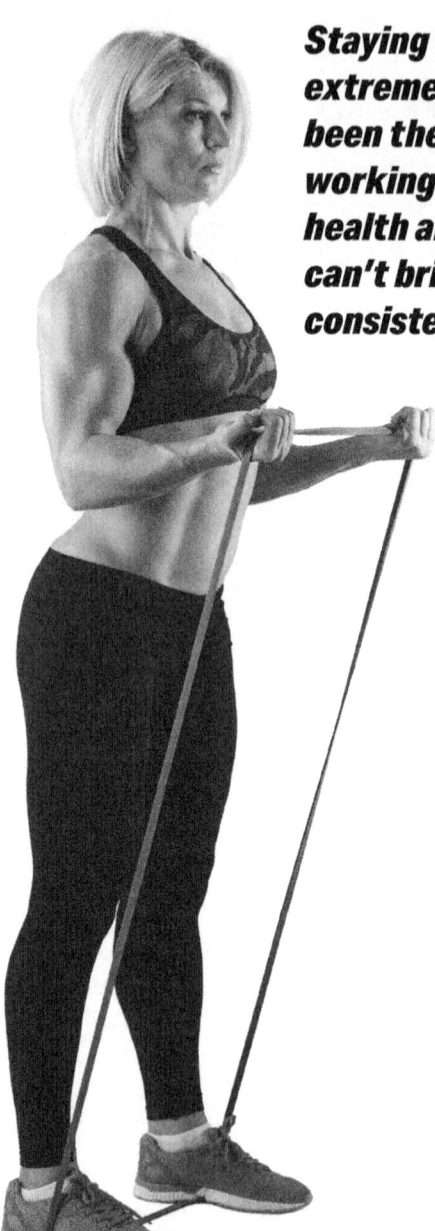

Staying fit can seem like an extremely daunting task. We've all been there, knowing that regularly working out will improve our overall health and wellbeing, but we just can't bring ourselves to start or be consistent with it.

Conventional methods of exercise, such as going to the gym, can be a bit of a hassle due to factors such as time, money, shyness, or lifestyle. This book is specifically designed to tackle this problem head-on, catering to people who are always busy, on the go, recovering from a recent injury, intimidated of working out at the gym, or simply don't want the inconvenience of having to pay for a membership. This book will provide exercises and tips on staying/getting in shape without even having to leave the comfort of your own home, only utilizing a simple piece of equipment, the resistance band.

Resistance training (also called weight or strength training) is a form of training that involves doing exercises that make the body do certain movements while trying to overcome external resistance (such as dumbbells, bodyweight, resistance bands, etc.). The repeated movements and resistance allow certain muscles to contract (depending on the exercise) and muscle fibers to be worn out. As a response, during rest, the muscles that were used regenerate to become bigger and stronger.

Resistance training is a vital part of any well-rounded exercise program. Besides improving muscle tone and strength, resistance training also reaps the following benefits:

- Promotes good balance, focus, and form
- Increases muscle-to-fat ratio
- Reduced risk of obesity and osteoporosis
- Improves mood
- Decreases blood pressure and cholesterol
- Improves cognitive function
- Decreases many types of chronic pain, such as arthritis, lower back pain, and fibromyalgia

Using a resistance band for resistance training, compared to going to the gym and using gym equipment, is a ton more cost-effective. This is because resistance bands are cheap and offer the benefit of a one-time purchase, in contrast to the regular rate of pay for a gym membership. Resistance bands also provide the versatility of being able to do exercises that target certain muscle groups while also taking up way less room than, say, if you buy your own gym equipment. This makes resistance bands a more portable, cheaper, and overall more convenient option for a busy schedule, especially while traveling.

CHAPTER 1:
RESISTANCE BANDS

What exactly are resistance bands? You have probably heard of or seen them before. They're training equipment that is primarily made of rubber or latex. Resistance bands may seem like a plain and simple tool; however, resistance bands can be used to execute a wide array of exercises. From shoulders, arms, abs, and even the whole body, resistance bands can train muscles just as effectively as dumbbells or gym equipment. Resistance band workouts can be done anywhere while still providing an effective workout. This is what makes them so effective and appealing to people who don't have the time or energy to go to the gym.

There are a plethora of different types of resistance bands, with each varying in length, width, and color. Their shapes and thicknesses may also be different from one another. Each type is best suited for a certain type of exercise, so it is important to remember to use each type how it was designed to be used. This maximizes your workout and helps prevent injuries. An outline of the most common types of resistance bands is listed below and which exercises they are mostly catered for.

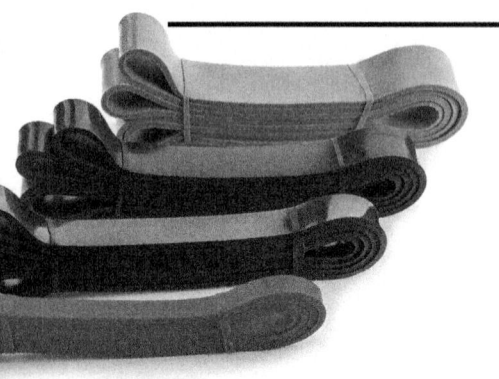

POWER RESISTANCE LOOP BANDS

Power resistance loop bands are long, thick bands that are characterized by their continuous flat loop. This band's massive size enables it to be used in a variety of exercises, making it one of the most versatile. There is an exercise for almost every muscle group that uses power resistance loop bands, so this item is a great first purchase if you are not able to buy every type at once. They are also called heavy-duty resistance bands.

MINI LOOP BANDS

Mini loop bands, as suggested by its name, are essentially shorter and wider power resistance loop bands. There are two common variants of mini loop bands: Plain rubber and non-slip. The main difference between the two is that non-slip mini loop bands have fabric covering the rubber/latex. This is added for comfort and the prevention of one's hands from rolling up. Mini loop bands are commonly used to train the lower body and are present in exercises such as squats, leg extensions, and glute and hip exercises. However, there are some upper body exercises that use mini loop bands as well.

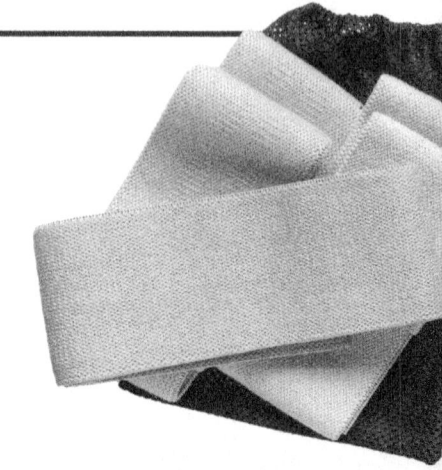

CHAPTER 1: RESISTANCE BANDS

TUBE BANDS

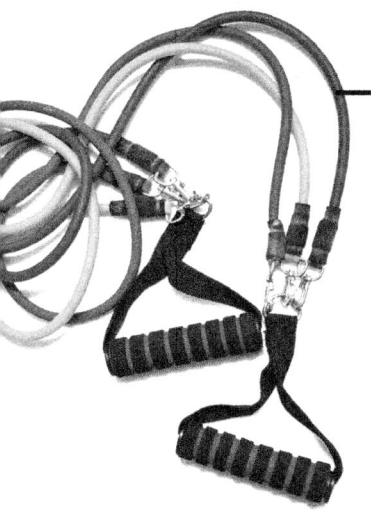

Tube bands are resistance bands characterized by the rubber's round shape and plastic handles attached to each end. They are commonly employed to mimic dumbbell and gym machine exercises like curls, shoulder presses, and back rows. This is done by being anchored or tied to doors, bars, and poles, among other things. Because of this, tube resistance bands offer great versatility for upper body training and are a good pair with mini loop bands. A session incorporating tube bands and mini loop bands will provide an effective workout for the entire body.

THERAPY BANDS

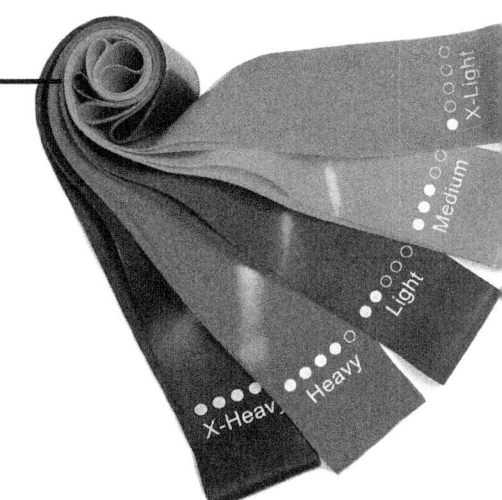

Therapy bands are long, thin, and flat resistance bands that are not looped or have any handles. Therapy bands are commonly used to treat people with injuries or people who are just recovering from them. The elderly can also utilize these bands for an effective, low-impact workout. Furthermore, therapy bands are very effective for stretching and can be used as a warm-up before an intense workout.

RESISTANCE BAND LEVELS

Many varieties of resistance bands have difficulty levels that correspond to their color. The power resistance loop band and mini loop band are common bands that are like this. Easier bands are usually thinner and easier to stretch, while more difficult bands are thicker, offering more resistance.

Having resistance bands of different levels is beneficial, as having different levels on hand enables one to do variations of many different exercises. The difficulty of an exercise can be made harder or easier by simply using a different band! Different brands have different levels. Some have 4 strength levels, while others can have up to 8 levels. Something that stays consistent within these brands is which color is assigned to each difficulty level. Most brands generally follow the order of yellow, red, green, blue, and black, with yellow being the easiest and black being the most difficult. Some companies may add other colors such as tan or pink, but memorizing the common colors should serve enough as a guide when purchasing a new resistance band.

CHAPTER 2:
GAUGING YOUR LEVEL

Knowing your boundaries, goals, and skill level is a vital part of fitness, no matter what equipment you're using. Knowing your own body's capabilities prevents you from injuries that will set you back in your fitness journey. Having a specific goal in mind will encourage motivation and provide a clear indication of progress.

Whether it be physically, mentally, or lifestyle-wise, everybody is different. Thus, one's goals and fitness level will most likely differ from others around them. There are many, many factors that may influence one's fitness level and objectives. Some examples are:

- Diet
- Fitness experience
- Time
- Priorities and values
- Medical conditions
- Gender
- Age

Below will go over some basic guidelines for the fitness levels of beginner, intermediate and advanced. It's important to carefully read over these so you can successfully find your fitness level.

BEGINNER

Someone who is at the beginner level of fitness generally has little to no experience in exercising regularly. Someone may also be at the beginner level if they are elderly, recovering from an injury, or severely out of shape, no matter their fitness experience. Because of this, it's important for beginners to start slow and work their way up. Beginners should find a resistance band that encourages them to use a good amount of force but shouldn't force them to struggle. It might also be beneficial for beginners to include more cardio in their workout routine if they are trying to lose weight and more strength training if they want to build muscle.

Frequency: 2-3 days a week, 20-30 minutes a session

Workout Intensity: low to medium-low

Example workout day:

Full body-choose 1-2 exercises from each section (chest, shoulders, core, etc.) and complete 2 sets of 5-10 reps for each exercise.

Muscle-specific-choose 5-8 exercises for each muscle you want to target. Complete 3 sets of 5-10 reps for each exercise.

CHAPTER 2: GAUGING YOUR LEVEL

INTERMEDIATE

A person at an intermediate fitness level will usually have a fair amount of fitness experience. They exercise regularly and will have most likely found their footing with exercise, doing some organized cardio/strength training here and there. They have learned the basics of sets, reps, and modifications. They are capable of utilizing the experience they have gained to stay fit and exercise according to their body's needs. Intermediate trainees have probably never had a strict workout schedule, have a difficult time staying consistent, or are still on the road to more advanced practices.

Consistency and willpower are what intermediate individuals have to have a lot of to pull through and be on their way to becoming advanced. Starting out in the middle difficulties of resistance bands would be a good idea. Once they have set out an adequate workout regimen and are staying consistent, they can take on the harder resistance bands and start getting ready for advanced exercises.

Frequency: 3-4 days a week, 40-60 minutes a session

Workout Intensity: Medium to high

Example workout day:

Full body-Choose 3-5 exercises from each section (chest, shoulders, core etc.) and complete 2 sets of 10-15 reps for each exercise.

Muscle-specific-Choose 7-10 exercises for each muscle you want to target. Complete 3 sets of 10-15 reps for each exercise.

ADVANCED

People at an advanced level of fitness typically enjoy hard, lengthy workout sessions and eagerly challenge their bodies to new lengths. They usually are already physically fit and have years of fitness experience under their belt. They know their own body's needs and are able to vary/adapt their workouts according to their schedule and constraints while still maintaining consistency and intensity. Their goal isn't to become fit anymore but rather stay fit or become even stronger.

Advanced individuals can take on the hardest leveled resistance bands and enjoy the challenge they will get. It's crucial for advanced trainees to change up their workouts every few months so that their body doesn't get used to their regimen and stop growing.

Frequency: 4-6 days a week, 60-90 minutes a session

Workout Intensity: high to very high

Example workout day:

Full body-Choose 3-5 exercises from each section (chest, shoulders, core etc.) and complete 3 sets of 15-20 reps for each exercise

Muscle-specific-Choose 10-all exercises in a section for each muscle you want to target. Complete 3 sets of 15-20 reps for each exercise.

CHAPTER 3:
BEFORE YOU BEGIN

This book is a guide containing all you need to know about resistance band workouts and resistance band exercises. This book will enable you to create an effective resistance training regimen that will allow you to stay fit. The most important word in that sentence is you. While the resources here are available for you to utilize, only you can push yourself to reach that goal of becoming/staying fit. It is absolutely crucial to remember to put in the utmost effort to pull through and not waste the labor you'll put into reaching your dream body. Try to stay consistent, and keep in mind that nutrition and diet are just as important (if not more important) than exercise. So pairing a resistance band training schedule with a balanced diet will be the key to success.

Below are a number of other important things to keep in mind regarding fitness:

STRETCHING AND WARMING UP

Warming up your body (through low-intensity exercises such as jumping jacks) before an intense workout will drastically improve performance. This is because warming up increases blood flow to muscles and loosens stiff joints, allowing muscles to carry out movements more effectively. Warming up is also important for preventing injuries, as a stiff body has a greater chance of being injured during physical activity than a warmed-up one.

A cool-down after a hard workout is also recommended, as this lets the body know that it is done and prepares it for growth and repair. A cool-down usually doesn't need to last longer than 5-10 minutes and just involves some deep stretching.

BREATHING

A common mistake that beginners and even some intermediates make is not breathing properly during exercise. People typically hold their breath to balance or to stabilize themselves. This is a bad habit, as muscles need oxygen to work properly. Not breathing will just make you end up being tired quicker and may even cause dizziness or muscle cramps. The best type of breathing is consistent, deep breaths for intense or prolonged exercises.

QUALITY OVER QUANTITY

Beginners often think that they need to work out for long, extended periods of time and have to do quick, burst-like movements to get as many repetitions as possible. This is not a good idea. It is better to have a slow, quick, high-quality workout than a long, low-quality one. Doing movements too much/quickly will mess up muscle contraction and, at best, kill gains, while at worst, cause an injury. Employ the speed and amount of repetitions that will challenge your body but won't make it too uncomfortable or especially hurt.

CHAPTER 3: BEFORE YOU BEGIN

PROGRESSIVE OVERLOAD

This may be a term that you've heard being thrown around before. Basically, progressive overload is the principle of gradually increasing your workout load to promote consistent growth in your muscles. Progressive overload is important as doing the same exercises at the same frequency, with the same weight for a long period of time, will make your body get used to it. This isn't good as the human body will not grow and become stronger if it's too comfortable, so progressive overload prevents this from happening by forcing the body to constantly adapt to overcome the greater load.

There are a number of ways to progressively overload. These can be increasing weight, frequency, repetitions, or decreasing rest time. But the technique you employ will fall in line with what kind of training you do. For example, an endurance runner will most likely employ the use of decreasing the rest time in between their runs so that their endurance doesn't plateau and will consistently get better. For resistance band training, employing progressive overload can be as simple as increasing the difficulty level of the resistance band you use overtime. Another effective progressive overload technique is to increase the length of your workouts. No matter what technique you choose, it's always beneficial to keep challenging yourself, no matter what fitness level you are!

BASIC GYM TERMS

Regardless of your fitness level, it's a good idea to know all the basic gym terminologies, as a lot of them will be used in this book, as well as in other situations in real life.

REPS: Reps are an abbreviation of the word 'repetitions' and are the number of times a certain movement is repeated. For example, fifteen banded shoulder presses mean doing the movement, banded shoulder presses, fifteen times.

SETS: A set is a name for the number of reps to be completed in a row before rest. Doing fifteen banded shoulder presses in a row, for example, is one set. Two sets of shoulder presses will incorporate thirty shoulder presses. There is usually a few seconds of rest between each set.

CARDIO: Cardio is an abbreviation for "cardiorespiratory" and includes exercises that increase heart rate, burning a sufficient amount of fat. Any exercise can be considered cardio as most exercises raise the heart rate. But when people talk about cardio, they are commonly thinking of exercises like swimming, running, or cycling.

UPPER BODY: Everything muscle above the belt. The chest, shoulders, triceps, biceps, back, and arms.

LOWER BODY: Every area below the belt. Thighs, glutes, legs, hamstrings, and calves.

CORE: The core houses all the muscles that make up the midsection of the body. This includes the famous six-pack.

RESISTANCE: This usually refers to the number of weight one's muscles are working against to complete a movement.

VARIATION: A variation of an exercise refers to a different way of doing it. Variations are employed to make an exercise either easier or harder.

CHAPTER 4:
HOW TO USE THIS BOOK

Creating a good workout routine that covers all the major muscle groups is crucial for effective muscular growth. This book will provide numerous resistance band exercises catered to the chest, shoulders, arms, back, legs, and core. The type of resistance band needed to carry out each exercise, as well as possible alternatives, will also be mentioned. You can create an entirely new workout plan using these exercises or even add them to your current one! An example of an effective resistance training regimen is the split system routine.

A split system routine aims to focus on one group of muscles each training session. This routine is effective as it provides sufficient attention to each muscle group while also giving them enough rest to recover and grow. There are different variations of the split system routine, with some being more specific than others. Some examples are shown below:

Monday-Upper body	Monday-Back and biceps
Tuesday-Lower body	Tuesday-Chest, shoulders, and triceps
Wednesday-Rest	Wednesday-Legs and abs
Thursday-Upper body	Thursday-Rest
Friday-Lower body	Friday-Back and biceps
Saturday-Rest	Saturday-Chest, shoulders, and triceps
Sunday-Cardio	Sunday-Legs and abs

Of course, you can decide which days you want to work out each muscle, as well as decide how many cardio and rest sessions there will be. You can even create a regimen for 2 weeks or decide on a different routine altogether. It all depends on your goals, and your body's needs, so it's important to take the time to create a routine that is suited for you! It might take some time, but once you've found a good routine, it's important to be consistent with it until you need to switch up.

There will also be variations included for each exercise that can be done if the exercise is too easy or too difficult. This is done so that each exercise can be included within every fitness level's workout routine, as well as provide a way to carry out progressive overload.

CHAPTER 4: HOW TO USE THIS BOOK

BASIC 5 MINUTE WARM-UP ROUTINE

We've already discussed the importance of starting each workout warmed up, so here's a quick full body warm-up routine that you can use before each workout:

JUMPING JACKS: -30 secs

PLANK: 30 secs

ARM CIRCLES: 30 secs forward, 30 secs backward

HIGH KNEES: 30 secs

WALK-OUTS: 30 secs

FRONT LUNGES: 30 secs

SQUATS: 30 secs

NECK ROTATIONS: 15 secs clockwise, 15 secs counter-clockwise

MOUNTAIN CLIMBERS: 30 secs

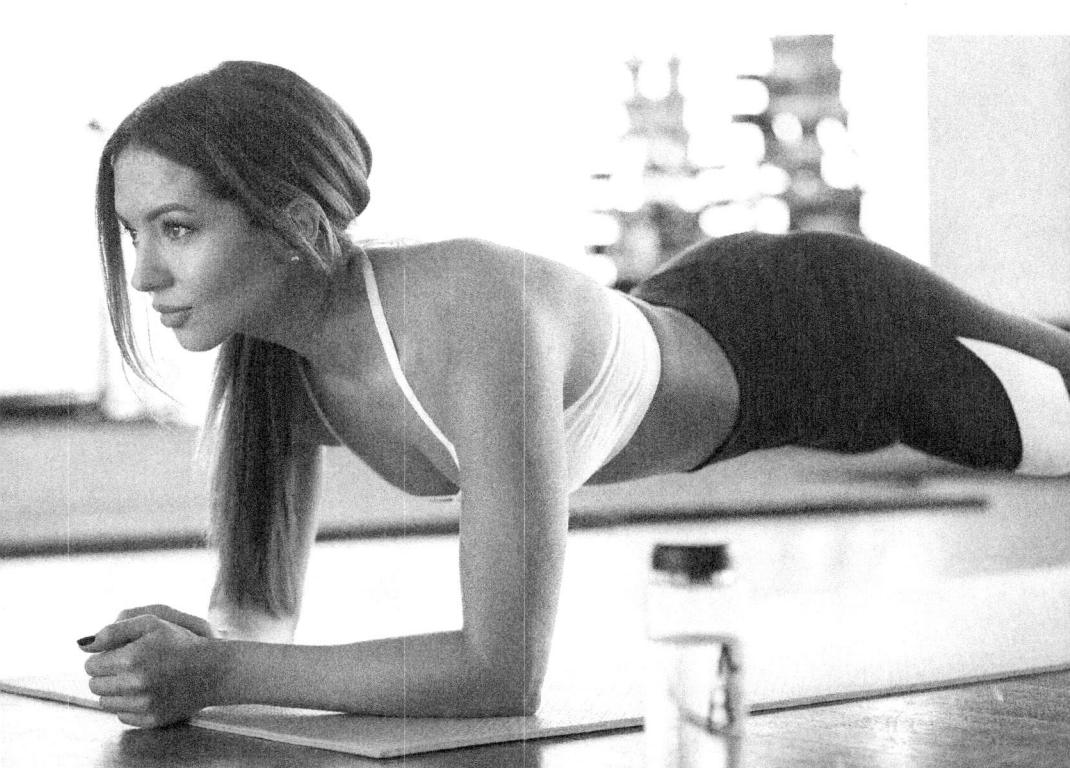

CHAPTER 5
CHEST

RESISTANCE BAND PUSH-UPS

RESISTANCE BAND REQUIRED: Power resistance loop band

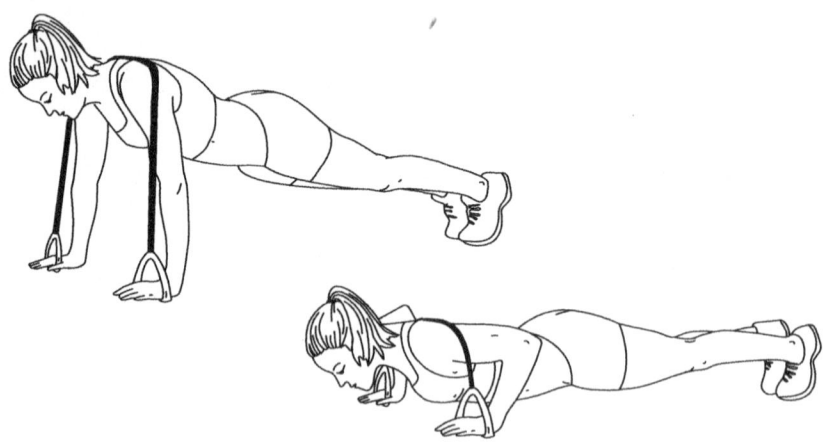

STEPS:

1 Place one end of the band on each hand between your thumb and index finger.

2 With your hands facing forward, lift the resistance band above your head and bring it down behind your back. Make sure the band is in line with your chest.

3 Get down into a regular push-up position, with the ends of the band secured under your palms. Go down slowly and push back up. Repeat for your desired number of reps.

VARIATIONS:

Easier-execute the exercise without a resistance band, only using bodyweight. An easier level of resistance band can also be used.

Harder-execute the exercise using a more difficult level of resistance band. Elevated or decline push-ups may also be done.

OTHER BANDS THAT CAN BE USED:

Tube band, therapy band-similar steps.

CHAPTER 5: CHEST

STANDING LOWER CHEST FLY

RESISTANCE BAND REQUIRED: Tube band

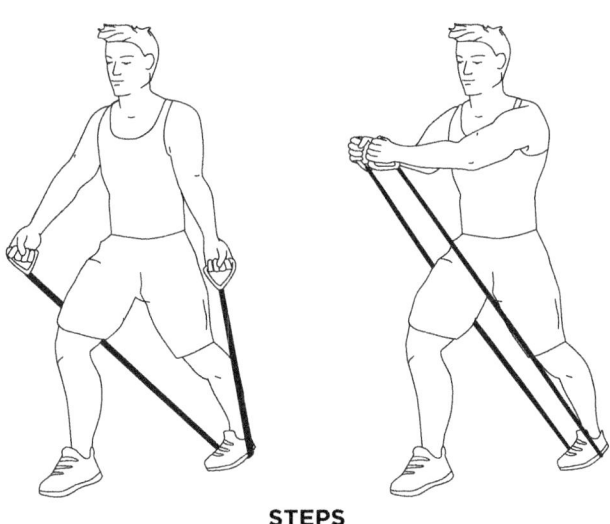

STEPS

1 Stand in a stance with one foot in front of the other stepping on the resistance band with the back foot.

2 For the starting position, grab both handles and hold them in line with your hips.

3 With a straight arm, lift the handles up to be in line with your face. Gently pull back down and repeat for your desired number of reps.

VARIATIONS:

Easier: Bring your feet closer together when stepping on the band to lessen resistance.

Harder: Bring your feet further apart when stepping on the band to increase resistance.

OTHER BANDS THAT CAN BE USED:

Power resistance loop band-step inside one end of the band and use the other end to pull up and down.

Therapy band-similar steps

CHAPTER 5: CHEST

RESISTANCE BAND CHEST PRESS

RESISTANCE BAND REQUIRED: TUBE BAND

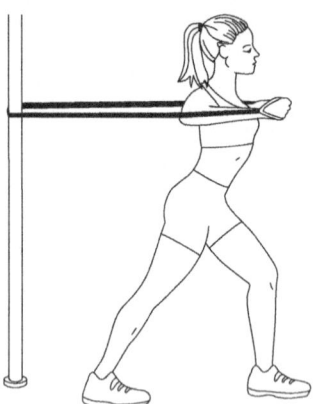
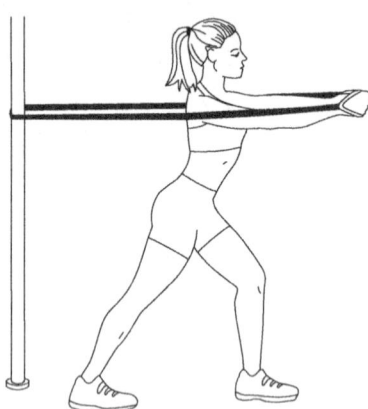

1 1Wrap the resistance band around an object that allows the band to reach chest level. Examples of this are a pole, high door handles, or a cupboard.

2 Take the handles and walk them out to a distance where a good amount of resistance is felt. Stand so that the band is behind you.

3 Hold the handles so that your knuckles are pointing up. Raise your hand to chest level and push out as far as you can, then return to the starting position. Repeat for your desired number of reps.

STEPS:
VARIATIONS:

Easier: Move back closer to the object the resistance band is wrapped around on. This decreases resistance.

Harder: Move further from the object the resistance band is wrapped around on. This increases resistance.

OTHER BANDS THAT CAN BE USED:

Power resistance loop band-similar steps.

Mini loop bands-Two mini loop bands are required for this method, as well as two different objects to wrap around (for each hand).

CHAPTER 5: CHEST

LYING CHEST PRESS

RESISTANCE BAND REQUIRED: MINI LOOP BAND

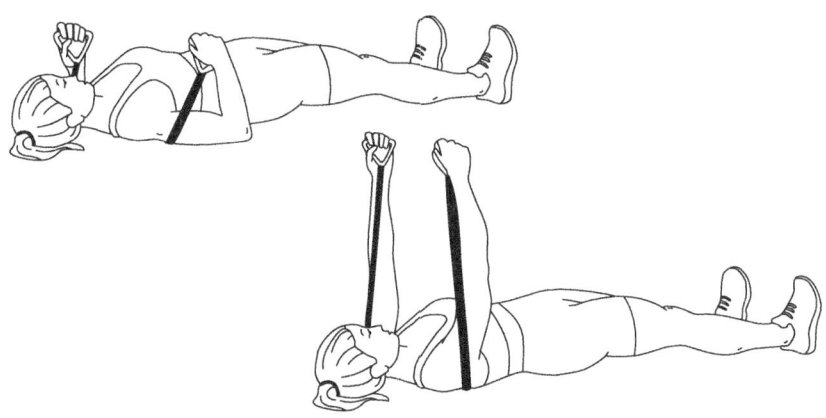

STEPS:

1 While lying down on a flat surface, wrap the band around your body in line with your chest. Legs should be bent.

2 Grab the end of the band that is over your body with knuckles facing down, hands apart.

3 Push up as far as you can, then bring back down. Repeat for your desired amount of reps.

VARIATIONS:

Easier: Perform the exercise using an easier level of mini loop band. Light household items like water bottles can also be used.

Harder: Spread your hands wider apart on the resistance band. This increases resistance.

OTHER BANDS THAT CAN BE USED:

Tube band, power resistance loop band, therapy band-these bands are significantly longer than the mini loop band. Because of this, each band has to be tied securely. Other than that, similar steps are followed.

CHAPTER 5: CHEST

LYING WIDE CHEST PRESS

RESISTANCE BAND REQUIRED: Power resistance loop band

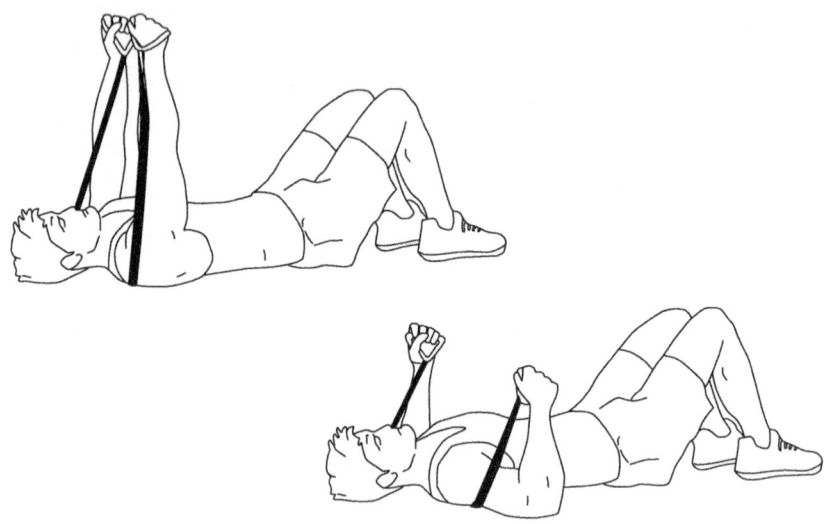

STEPS:

1. Lie down on a flat surface with your legs bent.
2. Grab the middle of the resistance band with both hands, ensuring that they are apart enough so when you pull, a good amount of resistance is felt. Knuckles should be facing back.
3. Lift the band straight up, then bring your elbows down, pulling the resistance band until your arms make a 90-degree angle. Bring back up and repeat for your desired number of reps.

VARIATIONS:

Easier: move your hands further apart when holding the band to decrease resistance.

Harder: move your hands closer together when holding the band to increase resistance.

OTHER BANDS THAT CAN BE USED:

Therapy band, tube band-similar steps.

CHAPTER 5: CHEST

LYING CRUSH PRESS

RESISTANCE BAND REQUIRED: Mini loop band

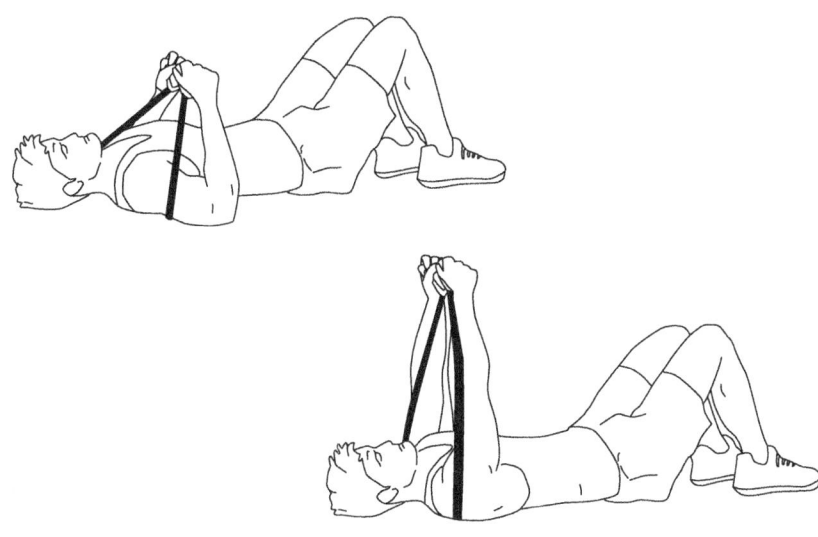

STEPS:

1 Lie down on a flat surface and wrap the band around your body, in line with your chest. Legs should be bent.

2 Grab the end that is over your body with both hands close together, knuckles facing outwards.

3 Push up as high as you can, then bring back down. Repeat for your desired amount of reps.

VARIATIONS:

Easier: execute the exercise using an easier level of resistance band.

Harder: execute the exercise using a more difficult level of resistance band.

OTHER BANDS THAT CAN BE USED:

Tube bands, power resistance loop bands, therapy bands-these bands are significantly longer than the mini loop bands. Because of this, each hand has to grab a shorter length. Other than that, similar steps are followed.

* *note that this exercise is different to the lying chest press, as this exercise targets more of the inner pecs, while the lying chest press targets the outer pecs.*

CHAPTER 5: CHEST

RESISTANCE BAND PULLOVER

RESISTANCE BAND REQUIRED: Therapy band

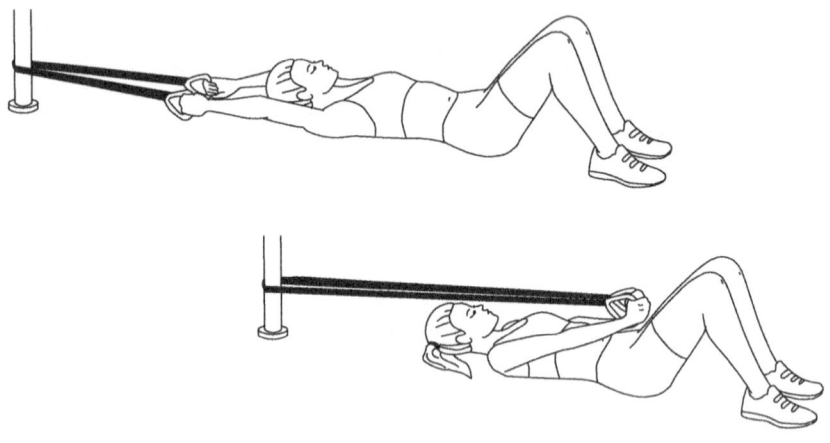

STEPS:

1 Secure the resistance band to an object that is low to the floor. Things like a table leg or pole should work well.

2 Lie on the floor, with the secured resistance band behind you. Grab the resistance band using both hands.

3 With straight arms, pull the band to be in line with your chest, then return to starting position. Repeat for your desired number of reps.

VARIATIONS:

Easier: Lie down closer to the resistance band and perform the exercise like that. The smaller distance decreases resistance.

Harder: Lie down further away from the resistance band and perform the exercise that way. The greater distance increases resistance.

OTHER BANDS THAT CAN BE USED:

Tube band-similar steps, but keep in mind that the handles may be an obstruction.

CHAPTER 5: CHEST

KNEELING BAND CHEST FLYS

RESISTANCE BAND NEEDED: Tube band

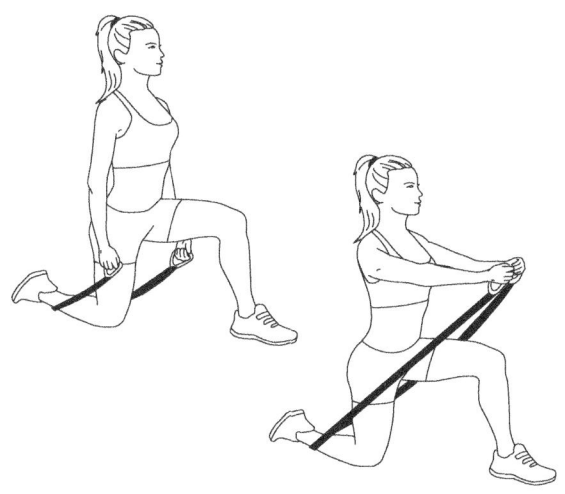

STEPS:

1 Kneel down with one leg in front and one at the back, both at about 90-degree angles.

2 Wrap the resistance band around the back leg, in between the foot and the knee.

3 Grab the handles and push out, then gently bring them back in. Repeat for your desired number of reps.

VARIATIONS:

Easier: Perform the exercise using a less difficult level of resistance band.

Harder: Ditch the handles and grab the band so that there is less distance between your hands and the anchor point. This increases resistance.

OTHER BANDS THAT CAN BE USED:

Therapy band, power resistance loop band-similar steps.

CHAPTER 5: CHEST

VALLEY PRESS
RESISTANCE BAND REQUIRED: Tube band

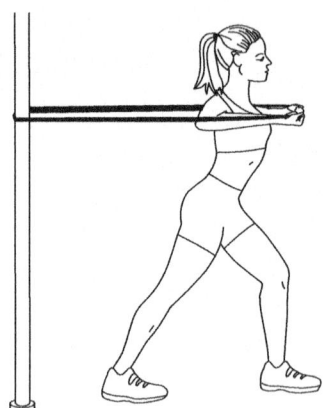 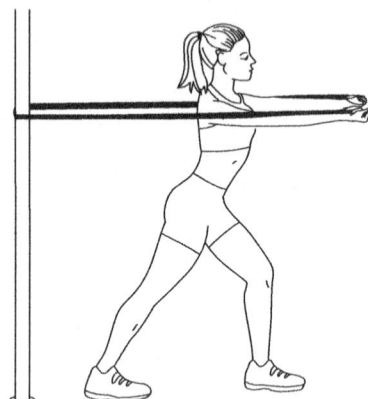

STEPS:

1 Wrap the resistance band around an object that allows the band to reach chest level. Examples of this are a pole, high door handles, or a cupboard.

2 Take the handles and walk them out to a distance where a good amount of resistance is felt.

3 Hold the handles so that the back of your hand is facing down. Put your hands together, then push out, then back in. Repeat for your desired amount of reps.

VARIATIONS:

Easier: Walk back closer to the object the resistance band is wrapped around on. This decreases resistance.

Harder: Walk further from the object the resistance band is wrapped around on. This increases resistance.

OTHER BANDS THAT CAN BE USED:

Therapy band, power resistance loop band-similar steps.

CHAPTER 5: CHEST

STANDING INCLINE WIDE FLY

RESISTANCE BAND REQUIRED: Therapy band

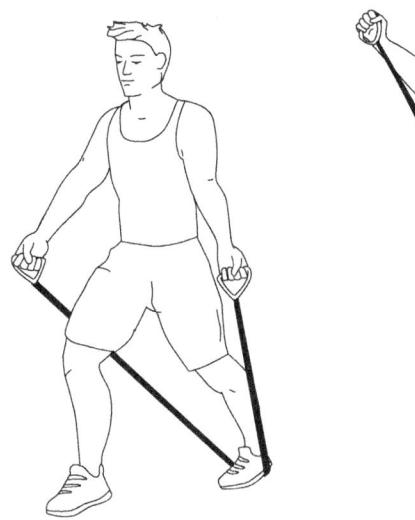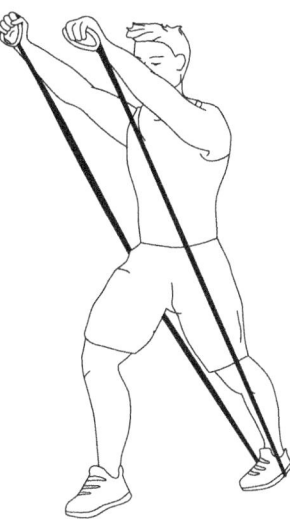

STEPS:

1. Step on the middle of the band with one foot.
2. Bring the foot with the band back, the other empty foot going forward.
3. Grab each end of the resistance band and hold them near your shoulders. Push up diagonally, then return back to the starting position. Repeat for your desired number of reps.

VARIATIONS:

Easier-bring your back foot closer to your front foot. This decreases resistance.

Harder-bring your back foot further from your front foot. This increases resistance.

OTHER BANDS THAT CAN BE USED:

Tube band, power resistance loop band-similar steps.

CHAPTER 5: CHEST

ALTERNATE CHEST PUNCHES

RESISTANCE BAND REQUIRED: Therapy band

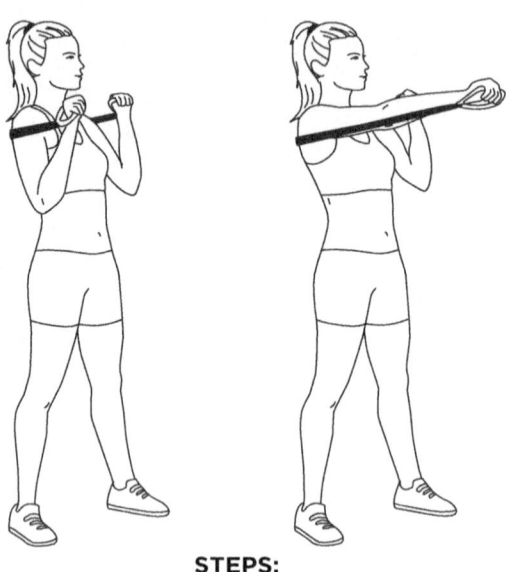

STEPS:

1. With your hands facing forward, grab each end of the resistance band and lift it above your head and bring it down behind your back, under your shoulders. Make sure the band is in line with your chest.

2. Wrap a little bit of the band around your wrist to a level that is comfortable.

3. Push one hand out like you're going for a punch, then push the other hand out while the other goes back to the starting position. Alternate/repeat for your desired number of reps.

VARIATIONS:

Easier-wrap less of the band around your wrist, decreasing resistance.

Harder-wrap more of the band around your wrist, increasing resistance.

OTHER BANDS THAT CAN BE USED:

Tube band, power resistance loop band-similar steps.

CHAPTER 6:
SHOULDERS

REVERSE FLYS

RESISTANCE BAND REQUIRED: Tube band

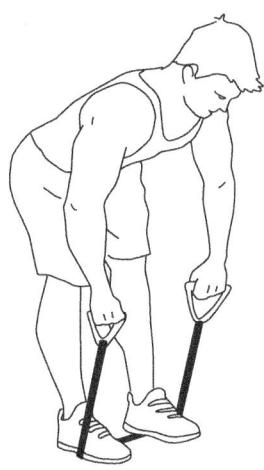 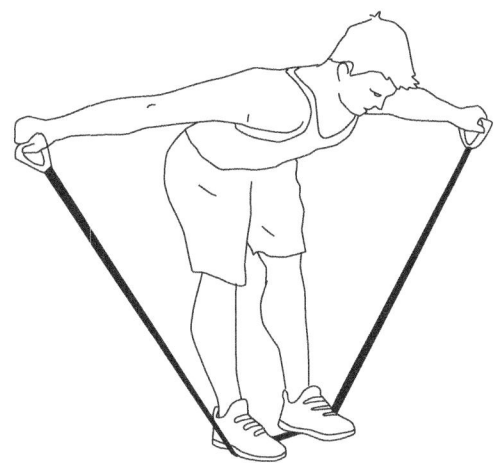

STEPS:

1 Step on the middle of the band with both feet.

2 Grab the handles, holding them up to about hip/upper thigh height with straight arms. Knuckles should be facing out to the side.

3 Lean forward slightly, then lift the handles outward, then upward. Pull up until in line with your shoulders. Remember to keep your arms as straight as possible. Repeat for your desired number of reps.

VARIATIONS:

Easier: Bring your feet closer together when stepping on the band to lessen resistance.

Harder: Bring your feet further apart when stepping on the band to increase resistance.

OTHER BANDS THAT CAN BE USED:

Therapy band, power resistance loop band-similar steps.

CHAPTER 6: SHOULDERS

FACE PULLS

RESISTANCE BAND REQUIRED: Power resistance loop band

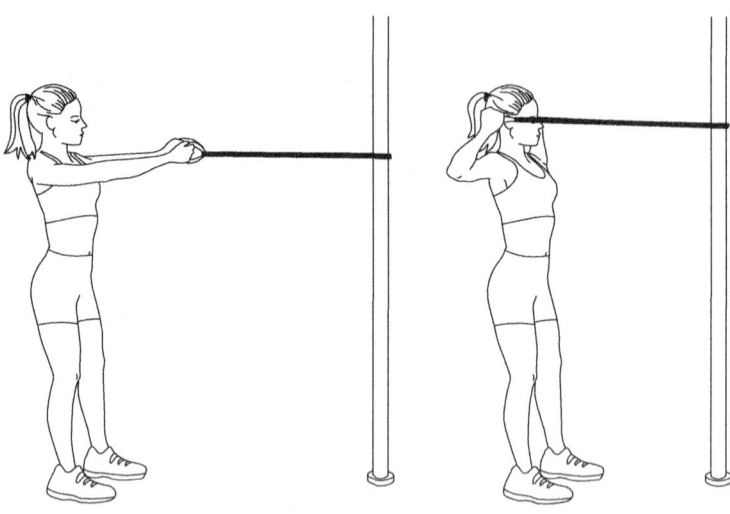

STEPS:

1 Tie the resistance band around any stable object that allows the band to be a bit below chest level. Examples of this are a pole, door handles, or table leg.

2 With the front of your body facing the resistance band, grab the end with both hands. Make sure your hands are a few inches apart. Walk the resistance band back to a distance that is comfortable.

3 To start, hold the resistance band with straight arms to about chest height, with knuckles facing up. Then, pull the band to be close to your face, with your elbows becoming in line with your shoulders. Return to the starting position and repeat for your desired number of reps.

VARIATIONS:

Easier: Walk closer to the object the resistance band is wrapped around on. This decreases resistance.

Harder: Walk further from the object the resistance band is wrapped around on. This increases resistance.

OTHER BANDS THAT CAN BE USED:

Therapy band, tube band-similar steps.

Mini loop bands-Two mini loop bands are needed for this method, as well as two different objects to wrap around. One band is possible, though, with one side being trained one at a time.

CHAPTER 6: SHOULDERS

OVERHEAD RAISE

RESISTANCE BAND REQUIRED: Tube band

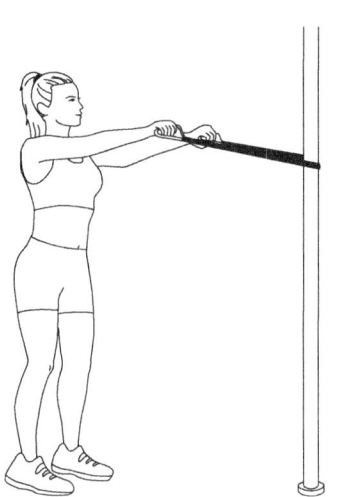 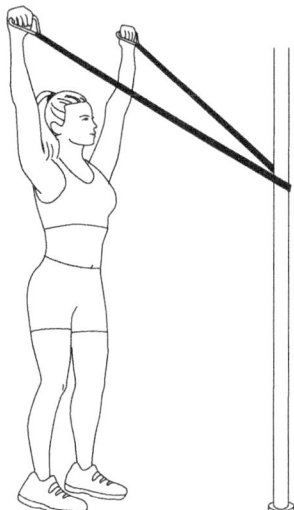

STEPS:

1 Tie the resistance band around any stable object that allows the band to be about chest level. Examples of this are a pole or door handles.

2 With the front of your body facing the resistance band, grab each handle with both hands, knuckles facing up. Walk the resistance band to a distance that is comfortable.

3 To start, hold the handles to about chest height. Then, with straight arms, pull/lift the handles to be directly over your head. Return to the starting position, then repeat for your desired number of reps.

VARIATIONS:

Easier-walk closer to the object the resistance band is wrapped around on. This decreases resistance.

Harder-walk further from the object the resistance band is wrapped around on. This increases resistance.

OTHER BANDS THAT CAN BE USED:

Therapy band, power resistance loop band-similar steps.

CHAPTER 6: SHOULDERS

FRONTAL RAISE

RESISTANCE BAND REQUIRED: Tube band

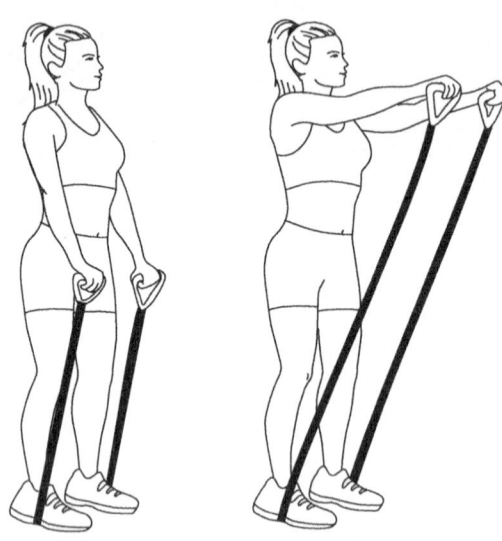

STEPS:

1 Step on the middle of the band with both feet.

2 Grab the handles, knuckles pointing up. Hold them to about hip/upper thigh height with straight arms.

3 Stand up straight, then pull the handles up until level with your face. Bring back down, then repeat for your desired number of reps.

VARIATIONS:

Easier-Bring your feet closer together when stepping on the band to lessen resistance.

Harder-Bring your feet further apart when stepping on the band to increase resistance.

OTHER BANDS THAT CAN BE USED:

Therapy band, power resistance loop band-similar steps.

CHAPTER 6: SHOULDERS

RESISTANCE BAND SHOULDER PRESS

RESISTANCE BAND REQUIRED: Tube band

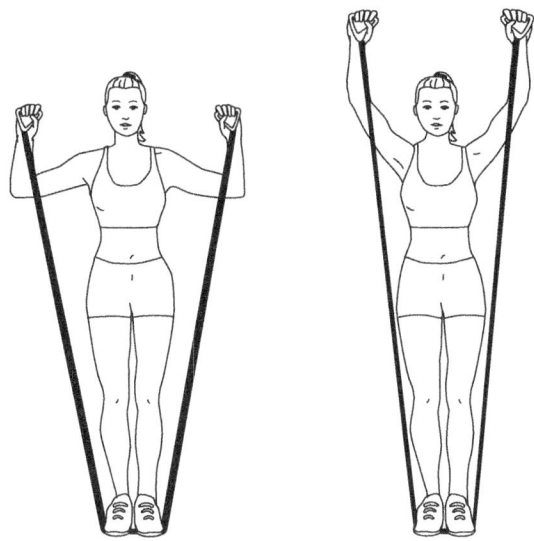

STEPS:

1 Step on the middle of the band with both feet.

2 To start, grab the handles and raise them up to be level with your shoulders. Hold the handles so that your knuckles are facing you and your arms are bent and facing up (like you're about to lift a box up that's on your head).

3 Pull the handles straight up, so they come above your head, return to the starting position. Repeat for your desired number of reps.

VARIATIONS:

Easier: Bring your feet closer together when stepping on the band to lessen resistance.

Harder: Bring your feet further apart when stepping on the band to increase resistance.

OTHER BANDS THAT CAN BE USED:

Therapy band, power resistance loop band-similar steps.

CHAPTER 6: SHOULDERS

LATERAL RAISE
RESISTANCE BAND REQUIRED: Tube band

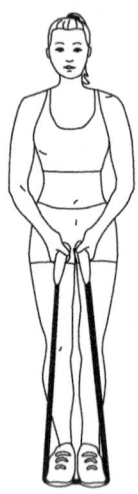
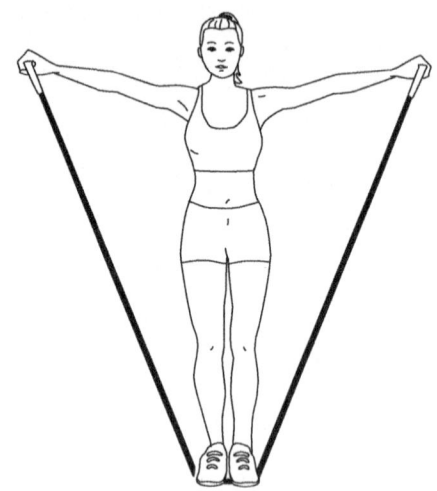

STEPS:

1 Step on the middle of the band with both feet.

2 Grab the handles and hold them so that your palms are looking inward, in line with your hips/upper thigh.

3 Stand straight, then lift both handles outward, then upward. Pull up until in line with your shoulders. Return to the starting position, and repeat for your desired number of reps.

VARIATIONS:
Easier: Bring your feet closer together when stepping on the band to lessen resistance.

Harder: Bring your feet further apart when stepping on the band to increase resistance.

OTHER BANDS THAT CAN BE USED:
Therapy band, power resistance loop band-similar steps.

CHAPTER 6: SHOULDERS

RESISTANCE BAND STRETCHES

RESISTANCE BAND REQUIRED: Power resistance loop band

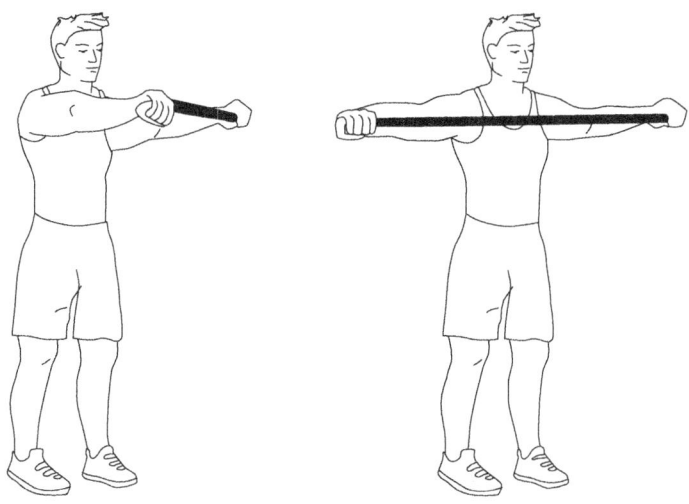

STEPS:

1 Grab the middle of the resistance band with both hands a few inches apart.

2 Lift the band in front of you, about in line with your chest.

3 With mostly straight arms, stretch the resistance band outwards with your hands as far as you can, without bringing your shoulder blades back. Return to the starting position and repeat for your desired number of reps.

VARIATIONS:

Easier: Move your hands further apart when holding the band to decrease resistance.

Harder: Move your hands closer together when holding the band to increase resistance.

OTHER BANDS THAT CAN BE USED:

Therapy band, tube band, mini loop band-similar steps.

CHAPTER 6: SHOULDERS

INTERNAL PULL-INS

RESISTANCE BAND REQUIRED: Power resistance loop band

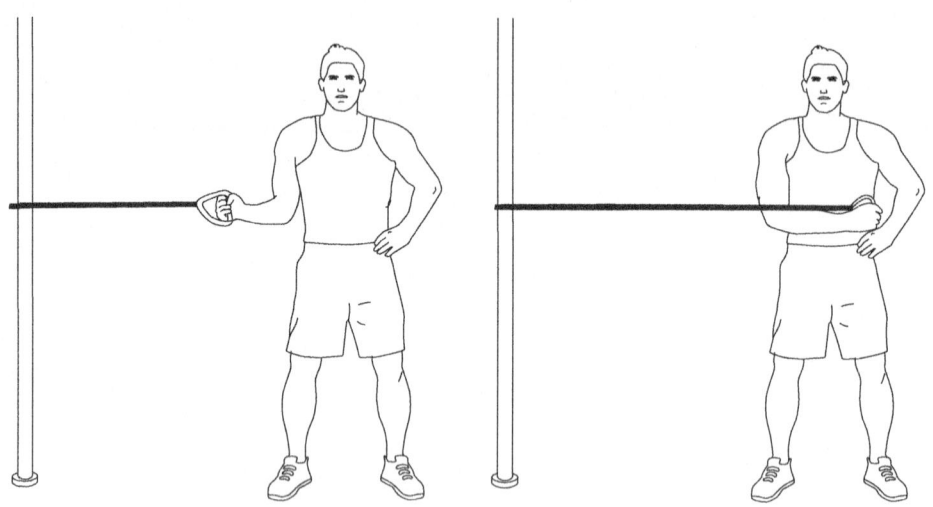

STEPS:

1 Tie the resistance band around any stable object that allows the band to be just slightly under chest level. Examples of this are a pole or door handles.

2 Stand sideways, then grab the end of the band with the hand closest to it. Hold it so that your arm makes a 90-degree angle, with your knuckles facing behind you. Walk the band out to a comfortable distance.

3 Pull the resistance band inward, up to your abdomen. Return to the starting position and repeat for your desired number of reps. Switch arms.

VARIATIONS:

Easier: Walk closer to the object the resistance band is wrapped around on. This decreases resistance.

Harder: Walk further from the object the resistance band is wrapped around on. This increases resistance.

OTHER BANDS THAT CAN BE USED:

Therapy band-similar steps.

Tube band-similar steps, with only one handle being used.

CHAPTER 6: SHOULDERS

EXTERNAL PULL-INS

RESISTANCE BAND REQUIRED: Power resistance loop band

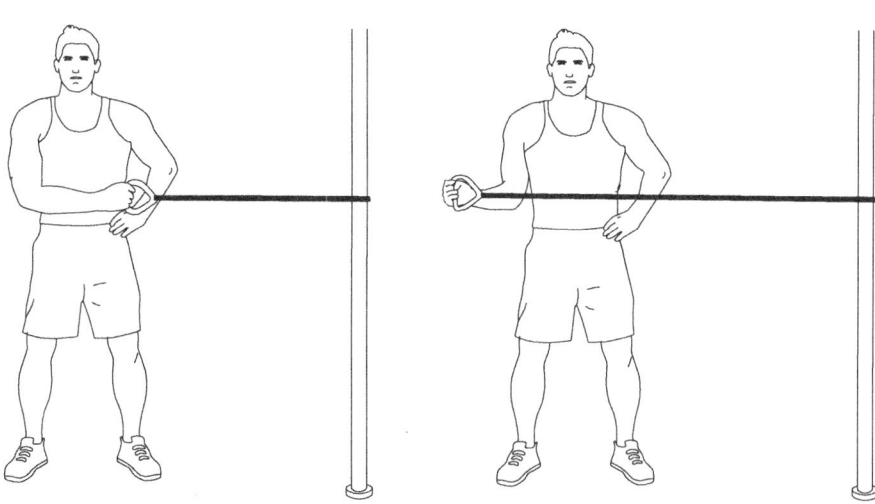

STEPS:

1 Tie the resistance band around any stable object that allows the band to be just slightly under chest level. Examples of this are a pole, or door handles.

2 Stand sideways, then grab the end of the band with the hand that's furthest from it. Hold it so that your arm makes a 90-degree angle, with your hands on your abdomen and knuckles facing forward. Walk the band out to a comfortable distance.

3 Pull the resistance band outwards as far as you can, then return to the starting position. Repeat for your desired number of reps.

VARIATIONS:

Easier: Walk closer to the object the resistance band is wrapped around on. This decreases resistance.

Harder Walk further from the object the resistance band is wrapped around on. This increases resistance.

OTHER BANDS THAT CAN BE USED:

Therapy band-similar steps.

Tube band-similar steps, with only one handle being used.

CHAPTER 6: SHOULDERS

PULL DOWNS

RESISTANCE BAND REQUIRED: Tube band

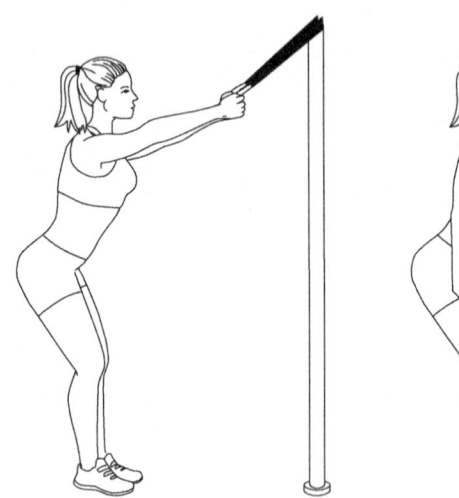 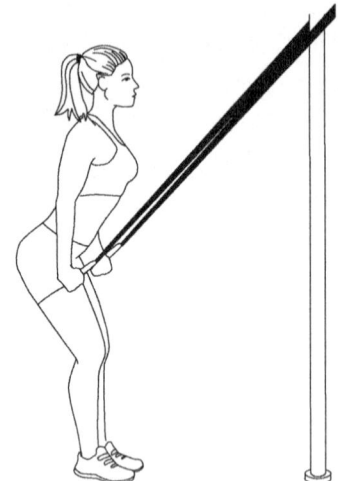

STEPS:

1 Anchor the resistance band over an object that is high above your head. Examples include a bar or a door. Make sure the band is anchored over evenly.

2 Grab both handles and hold them so that your knuckles face towards you.

Bend your knees to about a half squat and lean forward. Hold the handles level with your face, wide apart from each other.

3 Pull down on the handles as far as you can, then return to the starting position. Repeat for your desired number of reps.

VARIATIONS:

Easier:-ease your squat a little bit, or even just perform standing straight.

Harder:-ditch the handles and grip the band further up. This increases resistance.

OTHER BANDS THAT CAN BE USED:

Power resistance loop band, therapy band-similar steps.

CHAPTER 6: SHOULDERS

RECTANGULAR RAISES

RESISTANCE BAND REQUIRED: Tube band

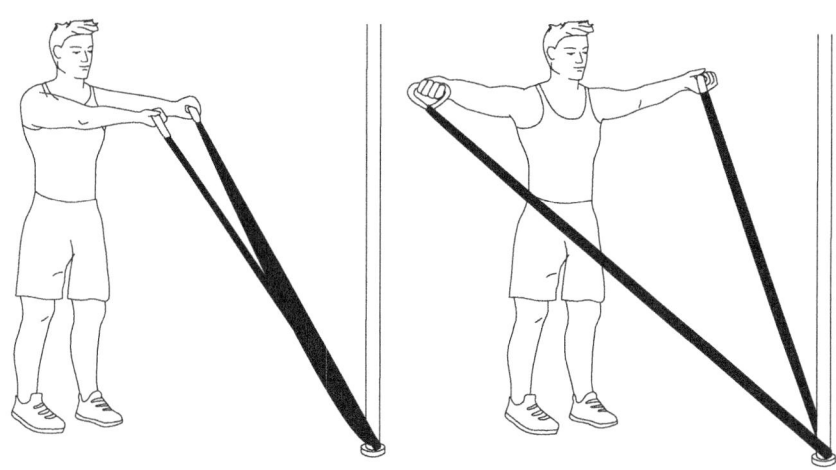

STEPS:

1 Wrap the resistance band around any stable object that allows the band to be low to the floor. A sturdy table leg or pole should do.

2 Grab both handles so that your knuckles are facing downwards. Walk the resistance band to a comfortable distance.

Start with the handles close together, about hip height. Then, lift them up all the way over your head.

3 From there, pull the handles outwards as far as you can, then bring each handle down, then back together again to the starting position. Repeat for your desired number of reps.

VARIATIONS:

Easier: walk closer to the object the resistance band is wrapped around on. This decreases resistance.

Harder: walk further from the object the resistance band is wrapped around on. This increases resistance.

OTHER BANDS THAT CAN BE USED:

Therapy band, power resistance loop band-similar steps.

CHAPTER 6: SHOULDERS

ONE ARM SKIS

RESISTANCE BAND REQUIRED: Power resistance loop band

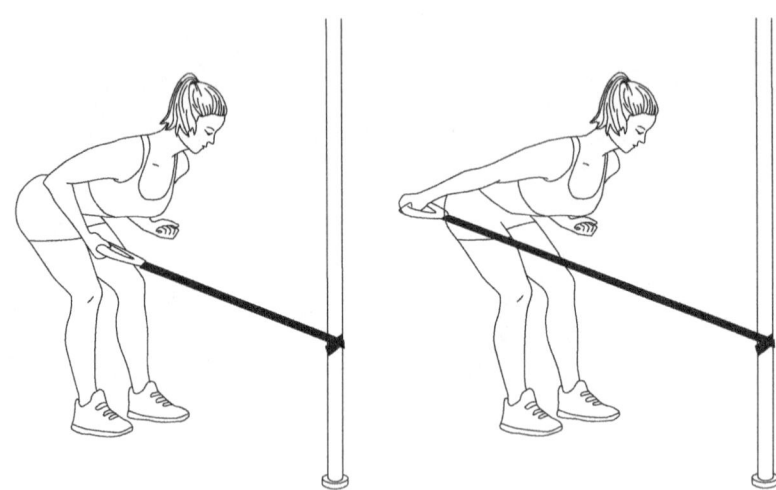

STEPS:

1. Wrap the resistance band around any stable object that allows the band to be low to the floor. A sturdy table leg or pole should do.

2. With the front of your body facing the band, grab the end with one arm, holding it so that your knuckles face outwards. Walk back a comfortable distance.

3. With feet shoulder-width apart, bend knees slightly and lean forward, holding the band in front. Then, with a straight arm, pull the band back as far as possible. Return the band in front of you and repeat for your desired number of reps.

VARIATIONS:

Easier: Walk closer to the object the resistance band is wrapped around on. This decreases resistance.

Harder: Walk further from the object the resistance band is wrapped around on. This increases resistance.

OTHER BANDS THAT CAN BE USED:

Therapy band-similar steps.

Tube band-similar steps, with one handle being used.

CHAPTER 7:
BACK

RESISTANCE BAND ROW

RESISTANCE BAND REQUIRED: Tube band

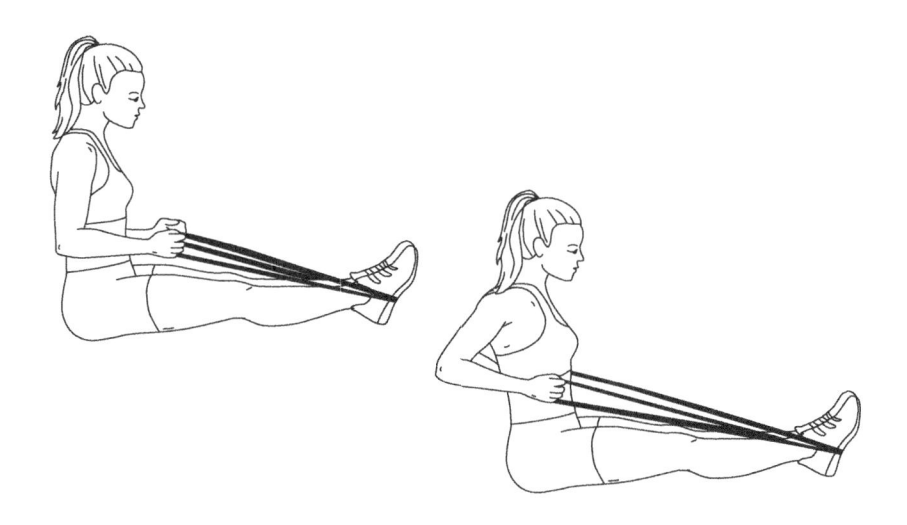

STEPS:

1 Sit down on a flat surface with your legs out and body at a 90-degree angle to your legs.

2 Wrap the resistance band around your feet.

3 Grab the handles so that your knuckles are facing out. Pull your elbows towards you, but don't bring your shoulder blades back. Slowly push back out. Repeat for your desired number of reps.

VARIATIONS:

Easier: Wrapping the band around only one leg will also make the exercise slightly easier.

Harder: Ditch the handles and grab the resistance band so that the distance between it and your hands is shorter.

OTHER BANDS THAT CAN BE USED:

Therapy band-similar steps.

Power resistance loop band-same steps, but since this band is longer, grabbing a shorter end is needed.

CHAPTER 7: BACK

BANDED BENT-OVER ROWS
RESISTANCE BAND REQUIRED: Tube band

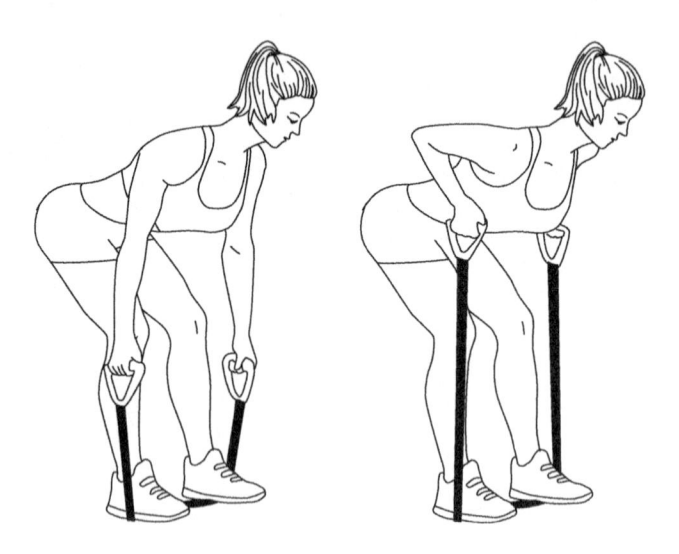

STEPS:

1 Step on the middle of the band with both feet, shoulder-width apart.

2 Grab the handles so that your knuckles are facing outwards. With straight arms under you, lean forward and slightly bend your knees.

3 Pull the handles up towards your chest until your elbows are ninety degrees. Gently bring the handles back down and repeat for your desired number of reps.

VARIATIONS:

Easier: Bring your feet closer together when stepping on the band to lessen resistance.

Harder: Bring your feet further apart when stepping on the band to increase resistance.

OTHER BANDS THAT CAN BE USED:

Therapy band, power resistance loop band-similar steps.

CHAPTER 7: BACK

BANDED BENT-OVER UNDER-HAND ROWS

RESISTANCE BAND REQUIRED: Tube band

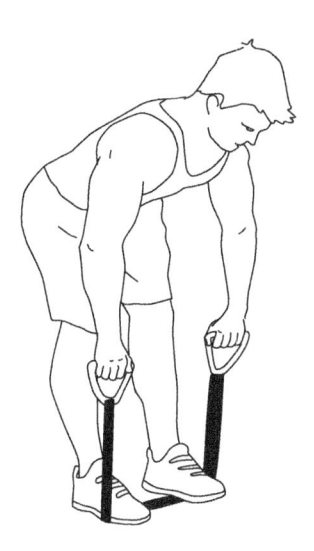

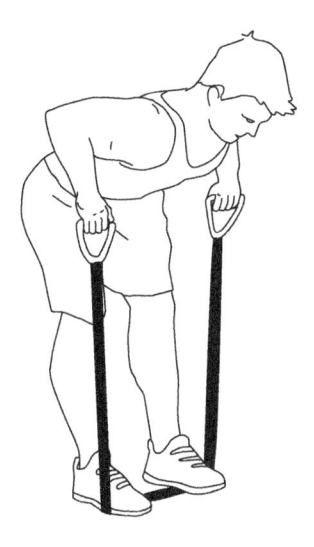

STEPS:

1 Step on the middle of the band with both feet, shoulder-width apart.

2 Grab the handles so that your knuckles are facing downwards. With straight arms under you, lean forward and slightly bend your knees.

3 Pull the handles all the way up towards your chest, bringing your shoulder blades back. Gently bring the handles back down and repeat for your desired number of reps.

VARIATIONS:

Easier: Bring your feet closer together when stepping on the band to lessen resistance.

Harder: Bring your feet further apart when stepping on the band to increase resistance.

OTHER BANDS THAT CAN BE USED:

Therapy band, power resistance loop band-similar steps.

CHAPTER 7: BACK

ELEVATED UNDER-HAND ROWS
RESISTANCE BAND REQUIRED: Tube band

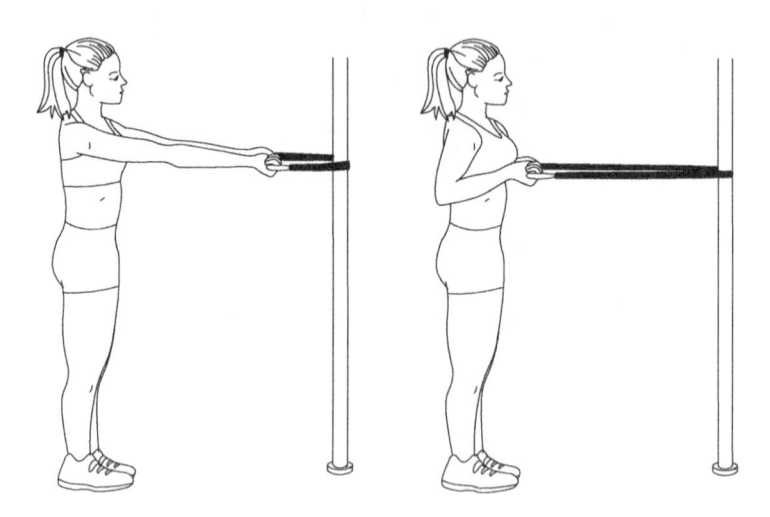

STEPS:

1 Wrap the resistance band around any stable object that allows the band to be about chest level. Examples of this are a pole or door handles. Facing the band, grab the handles so that your knuckles are facing downwards.

2 Walk the band to a comfortable distance, then kneel down with one leg at the front and one at the back. Make sure your legs form approximately 90-degree angles. Your arms should be straight out in front.

3 Pull the handles towards your chest, bringing your shoulder blades back. Return to the starting position and repeat for your desired number of reps.

VARIATIONS:

Easier: Walk closer to the object the resistance band is wrapped around on. This decreases resistance.

Harder: Walk further from the object the resistance band is wrapped around on. This increases resistance.

OTHER BANDS THAT CAN BE USED:

Therapy band, power resistance loop band-similar steps.

CHAPTER 7: BACK

ELEVATED ROWS

RESISTANCE BAND REQUIRED: Tube band

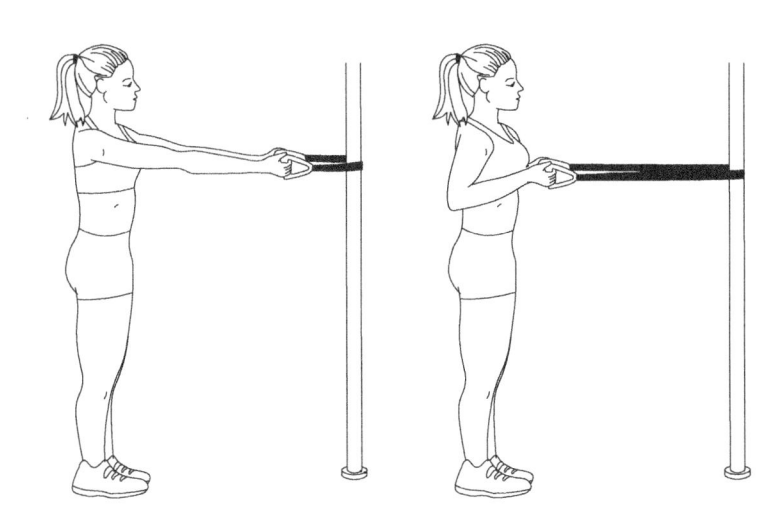

STEPS:

1 Wrap the resistance band around any stable object that allows the band to be about chest level. Examples of this are a pole, or door handles. Facing the band, grab the handles so that your knuckles are facing outwards.

2 Walk the band to a comfortable distance, then kneel down with one leg at the front and one at the back. Make sure your legs form approximately 90-degree angles. Your arms should be straight out in front.

3 Pull the handles towards your chest, bringing your shoulder blades back. Return to the starting position and repeat for your desired number of reps.

VARIATIONS:

Easier: Walk closer to the object the resistance band is wrapped around on. This decreases resistance.

Harder: Walk further from the object the resistance band is wrapped around on. This increases resistance.

OTHER BANDS THAT CAN BE USED:

Therapy band, power resistance loop band-similar steps.

* *Note that elevated rows and elevated under-hand rows are different exercises, like the different way of holding the resistance band allows different parts of the back to be hit.*

CHAPTER 7: BACK

REAR DELT PULL-OUTS

RESISTANCE BAND REQUIRED: Mini loop band

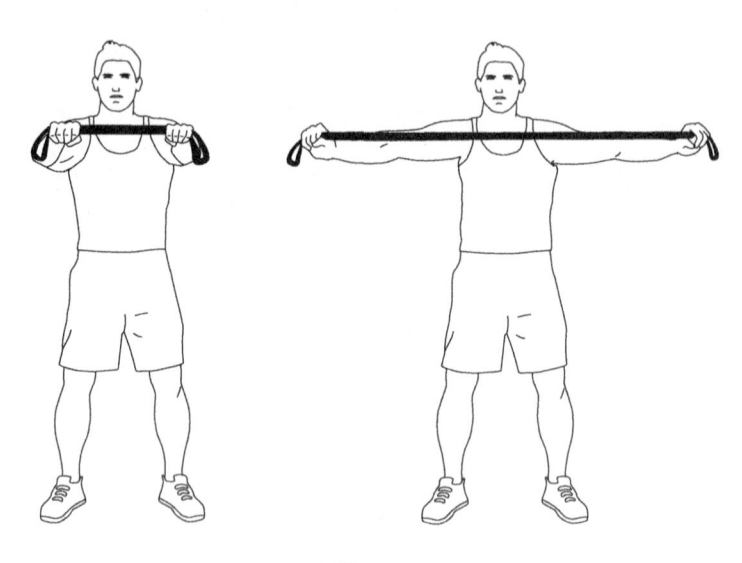

STEPS:

1 Put both of your hands flat on opposite sides inside the loop of the band, palms facing down.

2 While standing up, lift the band up with straight arms to about chest level.

3 Bend your elbows back as far as you can or until your shoulder blades meet. Return to the starting position and repeat for your desired number of reps.

VARIATIONS:

Easier: Perform the exercise using an easier level of resistance band.

Harder: Perform the exercise using a more difficult level of resistance band.

OTHER BANDS THAT CAN BE USED:

Therapy band, power resistance loop band, tube band-grab the middle of the band about a foot apart with a fist, knuckles pointing up. Then, perform as normal.

CHAPTER 7: BACK

ELEVATED STRAIGHT ARM PULLDOWNS

RESISTANCE BAND REQUIRED: Power resistance loop band

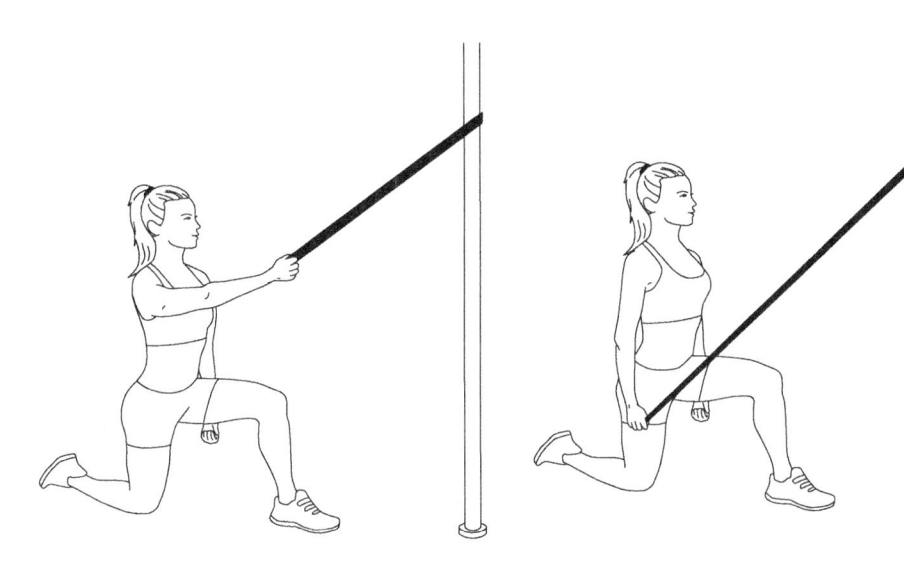

STEPS:

1 Tie the resistance band around any stable object that allows the band to be about chest level. Examples of this are a pole, high door handles, or a cupboard.

2 Take the handles and walk them out to a distance where a good amount of resistance is felt. Stand so that your side is facing the resistance band.

Kneel down with one leg in front and one at the back, both at about 90-degree angles.

3 Grab the end of the band with the arm closest to it and raise it up above your head. Your palms should be facing you.

Pull the band down to about hip level. Return to the starting position and repeat for your desired number of reps. Switch sides.

VARIATIONS:

Easier: Walk back closer to the object the resistance band is wrapped around on. This decreases resistance.

Harder: Walk further from the object the resistance band is wrapped around on. This increases resistance.

OTHER BANDS THAT CAN BE USED:

Therapy band, tube band-similar steps. If using the tube band, only use one of the handles.

CHAPTER 7: BACK

ELEVATED SIDE-ARM PULLDOWNS

RESISTANCE BAND REQUIRED: Power resistance loop band

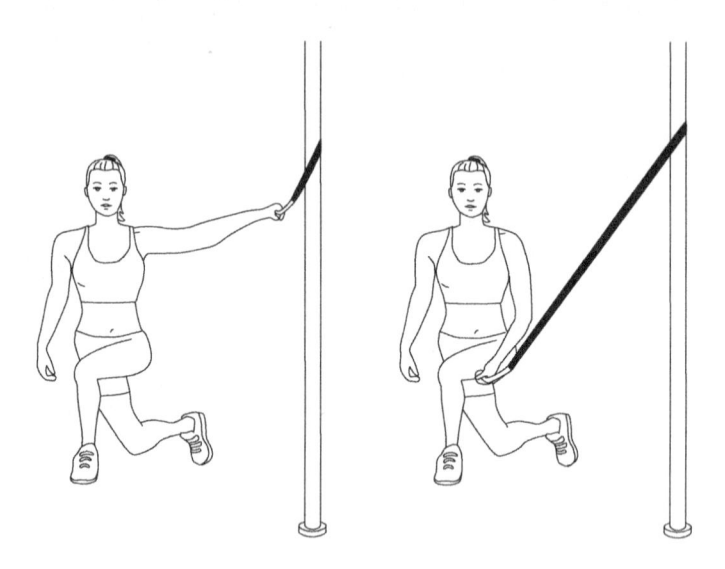

STEPS:

1 Tie the resistance band around any stable object that allows the band to be about chest level. Examples of this are a pole, high door handles or a cupboard.

2 Take the handles and walk them out to a distance where a good amount of resistance is felt. Stand so that your side is facing the resistance band.

Kneel down with one leg in front and one at the back, both at about 90-degree angles. Hold the band so that your knuckles are facing down.

3 To start, raise the band up above and to the side of your head with the arm closest to it. Then, bend your elbows down as far as you can. Return to the starting position and repeat for your desired number of reps. Switch sides.

VARIATIONS:

Easier: Move back closer to the object the resistance band is wrapped around on. This decreases resistance.

Harder: Move further from the object the resistance band is wrapped around on. This increases resistance.

OTHER BANDS THAT CAN BE USED:

Therapy band, tube band-similar steps. If using the tube band, only use one of the handles.

CHAPTER 7: BACK

BANDED ROMANIAN DEADLIFT

RESISTANCE BAND REQUIRED: Tube band

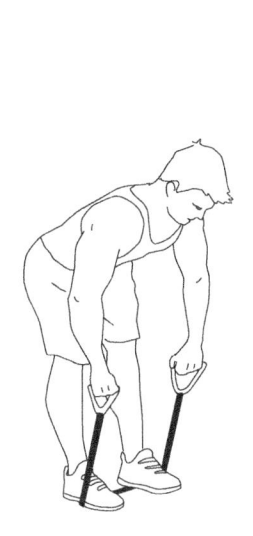

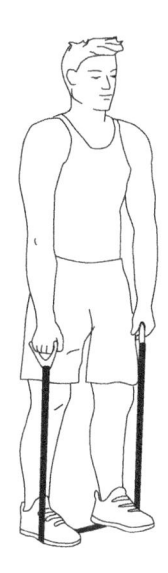

STEPS:

1 Step on the middle of the band with both feet.

2 Grab both handles so that your knuckles are facing away from you, at about hip height. Your hands should be in front of you.

3 With a straight back, lean forward until you feel a burn in your hamstrings. Hold for a second and then stand back up straight. Repeat for your desired number of reps.

VARIATIONS:

Easier: Bring your feet closer together when stepping on the band to lessen resistance.

Harder: Bring your feet further apart when stepping on the band to increase resistance.

OTHER BANDS THAT CAN BE USED:

Therapy band, power resistance loop band-similar steps.

CHAPTER 7: BACK

SINGLE-ARM ROWS

RESISTANCE BAND REQUIRED: Power resistance band

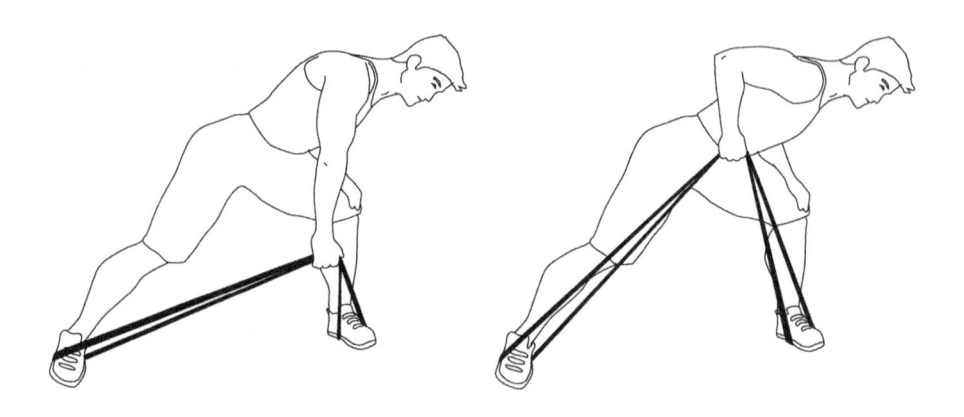

STEPS:

1 Step on each end of the resistance band with one foot in front of the other.

2 Grab the resistance band at the middle point between your front and back foot with one arm, knuckles pointing out. Arms should be straight at about hip height.

3 Bend over slightly, then pull your elbow back as far as you can. Bring back down and repeat for your desired number of reps. Switch arms.

VARIATIONS:

Easier: Bring your feet closer together, this creates less resistance.

Harder: Rather than stepping on the ends of the resistance band, step 10cm in from the ends, this creates more resistance.

OTHER BANDS THAT CAN BE USED:

Therapy band, Tube band -similar steps.

CHAPTER 7: BACK

BENT-OVER BACK FLYS

RESISTANCE BAND REQUIRED: Tube band

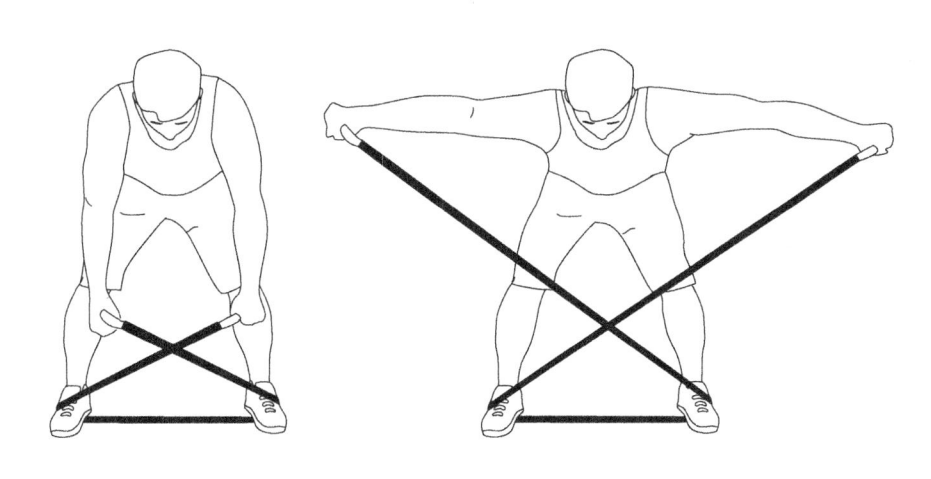

STEPS:

1 Step on the middle of the band with both feet. Cross each handle to the other side so that when lifted, the band forms an 'x.'

2 Grab the handles so that your knuckles are facing out, about hip height. Bend over to make an approximate 45-degree angle.

3 To start, put your hands together below you, with straight arms. Then, with slightly bent elbows, move the handles outwards, then upwards, until in line with your shoulders. Bring back to the starting position and repeat for your desired number of reps.

VARIATIONS:

Easier: Bring your feet closer together when stepping on the band to lessen resistance.

Harder: Bring your feet further apart when stepping on the band to increase resistance.

OTHER BANDS THAT CAN BE USED:

Therapy band, power resistance loop band-similar steps.

CHAPTER 7: BACK

SEATED PRONATED ROWS

RESISTANCE BAND REQUIRED: Tube band

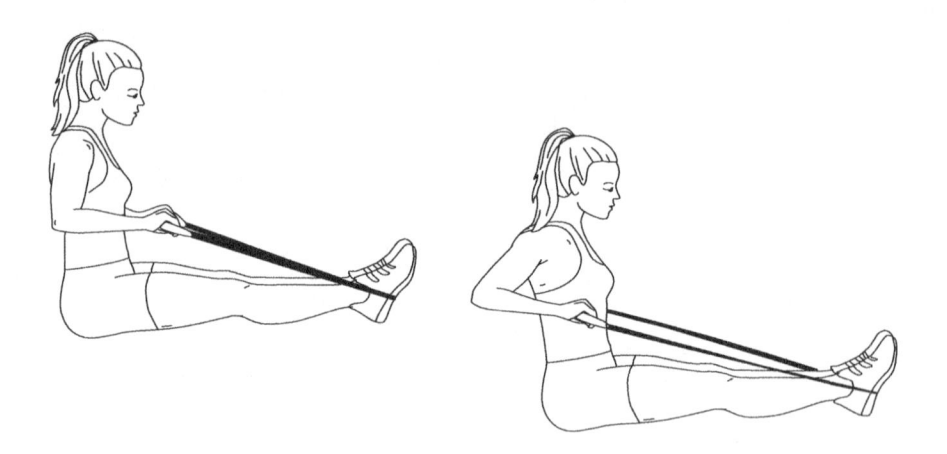

STEPS:

1 Sit down on a flat surface with your legs out and body at a 90-degree angle to your legs.

2 Wrap the resistance band around your feet. Grab the handles so that your knuckles are pointing up.

To start, have your arms straight in front of you, with your hands close

3 together. Then, bring the handles up to your chest, bending your shoulder blades back. Return to the starting position and repeat for your desired number of reps.

VARIATIONS:

Easier: Wrapping the band around only one leg will also make the exercise slightly easier.

Harder: Ditch the handles and grab the resistance band so that the distance between it and your hands is shorter.

OTHER BANDS THAT CAN BE USED:

Therapy band, power resistance loop band-similar steps.

CHAPTER 7: BACK

SEATED REVERSE ROWS
RESISTANCE BAND REQUIRED: Tube band

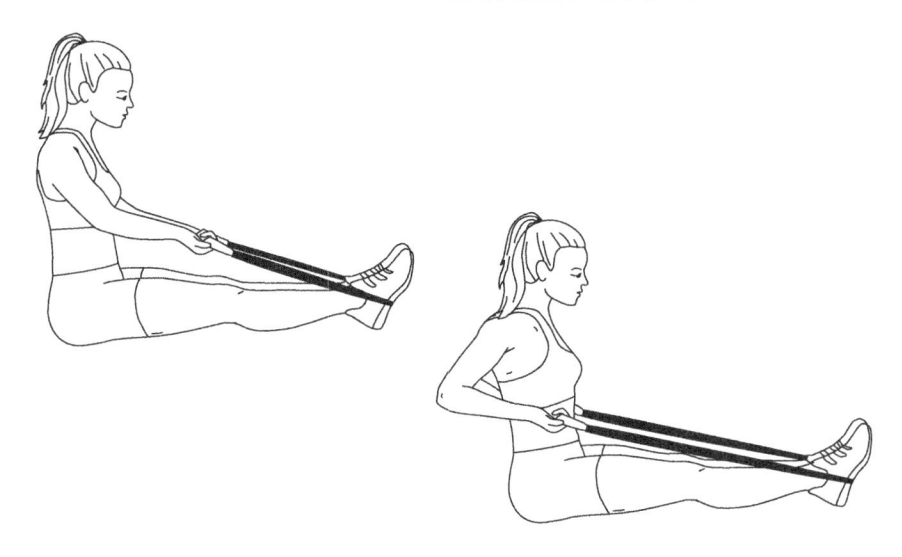

STEPS:

1 Sit down on a flat surface with your legs out and body at a 90-degree angle to your legs.

2 Wrap the resistance band around your feet. Grab the handles so that your knuckles are pointing down.

3 To start, have your arms straight, low, and in front of you, with your hands close together. Then, bring the handles to your hips, bending your shoulder blades back. Return to the starting position and repeat for your desired number of reps.

VARIATIONS:

Easier: Wrapping the band around only one leg will also make the exercise slightly easier.

Harder: Ditch the handles and grab the resistance band so that the distance between it and your hands is shorter.

OTHER BANDS THAT CAN BE USED:

Therapy band, power resistance loop band-similar steps.

CHAPTER 7: BACK

BANDED TRAP SHRUGS

RESISTANCE BAND REQUIRED: Power resistance loop band

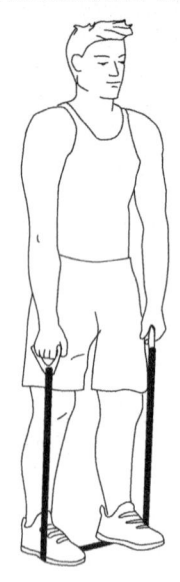

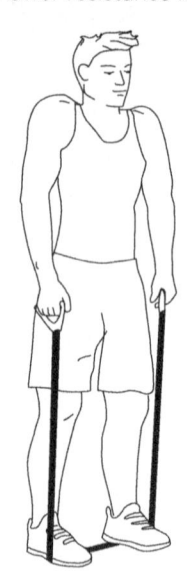

STEPS:

1 Step on the middle of the band with both feet.

2 Grab a bit further down the band until a good amount of resistance is felt. Your knuckles should be facing out to the side.

3 Lift your shoulders up to shrug, hold for a couple of seconds, then bring back down. Repeat for your desired number of reps.

VARIATIONS:

Easier: Bring your feet closer together when stepping on the band to lessen resistance. You can also grab further up the band

Harder: Bring your feet further apart when stepping on the band to increase resistance. You can also grab further down the band

OTHER BANDS THAT CAN BE USED:

Tube band, therapy band-similar steps.

CHAPTER 8:
ARMS

BANDED PUSH DOWNS-TRICEPS

RESISTANCE BAND REQUIRED: Power resistance loop band

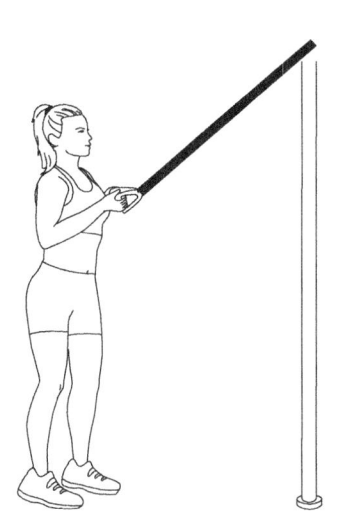

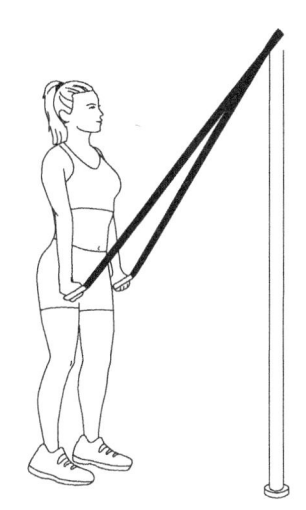

STEPS:

1 Tie one end of the resistance band around a stable, high anchor point. Examples of this are a pole or bar.

Grab the hanging end with two hands, knuckles facing outwards.

2 To start, bend your arms all the way up, elbows tight to your body.

3 Pull the resistance band down until your arms become straight, ensuring that your elbows stay still, with your hands doing all the pulling. Bring back to the starting position and repeat for your desired number of reps.

VARIATIONS:

Easier: Grab the band further down, up to the very end of the hanging end of the band. This decreases resistance.

Harder: Grab the band further up. This increases resistance

OTHER BANDS THAT CAN BE USED:

Tube band, therapy band-similar steps.

CHAPTER 8: ARMS

BANDED TRICEP EXTENSIONS-TRICEPS
RESISTANCE BAND REQUIRED: Tube band

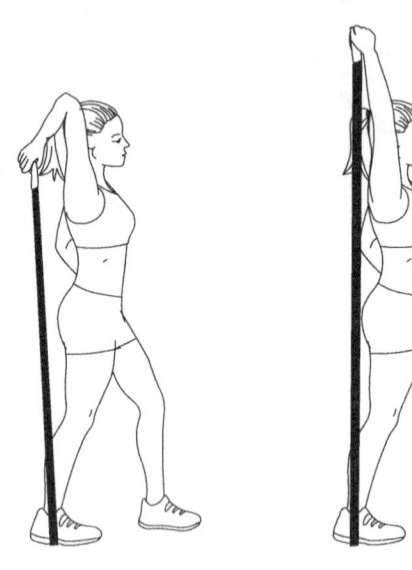

STEPS:

1 Step on the band with one foot, bringing the other foot slightly forward.

2 Grab the handles; lift all the way up so that they are behind your head. Your elbows should be facing forward, close to your ears.

3 Lift the handles up as far as you can, then bring them back to the starting position. Repeat for your desired number of reps.

VARIATIONS:
Easier-perform the exercise using a less difficult level of resistance band.
Harder-ditch the handles and grab further down. This increases resistance.

OTHER BANDS THAT CAN BE USED:
Therapy band, power resistance loop band-similar steps.

CHAPTER 8: ARMS

BANDED PULLBACKS-TRICEPS

RESISTANCE BAND REQUIRED: Tube band

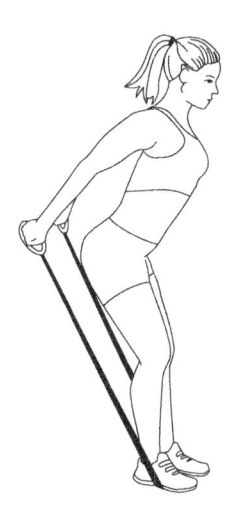

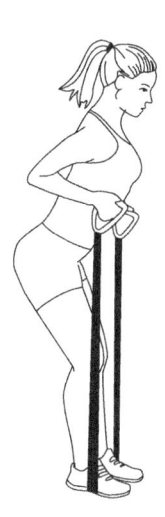

STEPS:

1. Step on the middle of the band with both feet.
2. Grab the handles so that your knuckles are facing forward, at about hip height. Bend forward at approximately a 45-degree angle.
3. Bring both handles up so that your arms are bent. Then, bring the handles all the way back using your arms until your arms become straight. Return back to the starting position and repeat for your desired number of reps.

VARIATIONS:

Easier: Bring your feet closer together when stepping on the band to lessen resistance.

Harder: Bring your feet further apart when stepping on the band to increase resistance.

OTHER BANDS THAT CAN BE USED:

Therapy band, power resistance loop band-similar steps.

CHAPTER 8: ARMS

SIDE SINGLE-ARM EXTENSIONS-TRICEPS

RESISTANCE BAND REQUIRED: Power resistance loop band

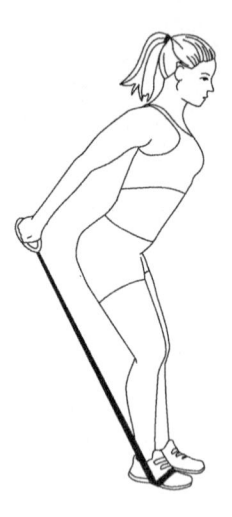

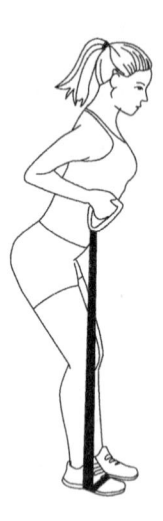

STEPS:

1. Step on one end of the band with one foot.

2. Grab the other end of the resistance band so that your knuckles are facing forward, at about hip height. Bend forward at approximately a 45-degree angle.

3. Bring the other end of the resistance band up so that your arm is bent. Then kick the hand holding the resistance band all the way back until your arms become straight. Return back to the starting position and repeat for your desired number of reps.

VARIATIONS:

Easier: Try not bending over as far while not kicking the arm back as high. However try to keep that arm as straight as possible in the contracted position.

Harder: Rather than stepping on the end of the resistance band, step 10cm in. This will create more resistance.

OTHER BANDS THAT CAN BE USED:

Tube band, therapy band-similar steps. When using the tube band, only use one handle.

CHAPTER 8: ARMS

MINI BANDED PULL DOWNS-TRICEPS

RESISTANCE BAND REQUIRED: Mini loop band

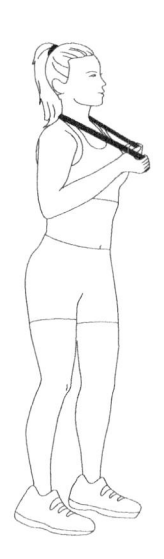

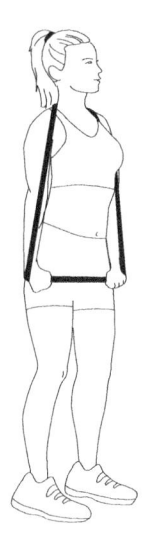

STEPS:

1 Stand with your feet slightly apart. Wear the band around one shoulder, like you would wearing a shoulder bag. Have the opposite hand between your shoulder and the band.

2 Hold the bottom end of the bend with the other free hand, knuckles pointing outwards. Start with your arm at about a 90-degree angle.

3 Pull the resistance band down until your arm is straight, then slowly bring it back up. Repeat for your desired number of reps. Switch arms.

VARIATIONS:

Easier: Perform the exercise using a less difficult level of resistance band.

Harder: Grab the resistance band further up. This increases resistance.

OTHER BANDS THAT CAN BE USED:

Therapy band, power resistance loop band, tube band-since these bands are significantly longer, they need to be wrapped/tied around your shoulders a number of times.

CHAPTER 8: ARMS

BANDED CLOSE GRIP PUSH-UPS-TRICEPS

RESISTANCE BAND REQUIRED: Power resistance loop band

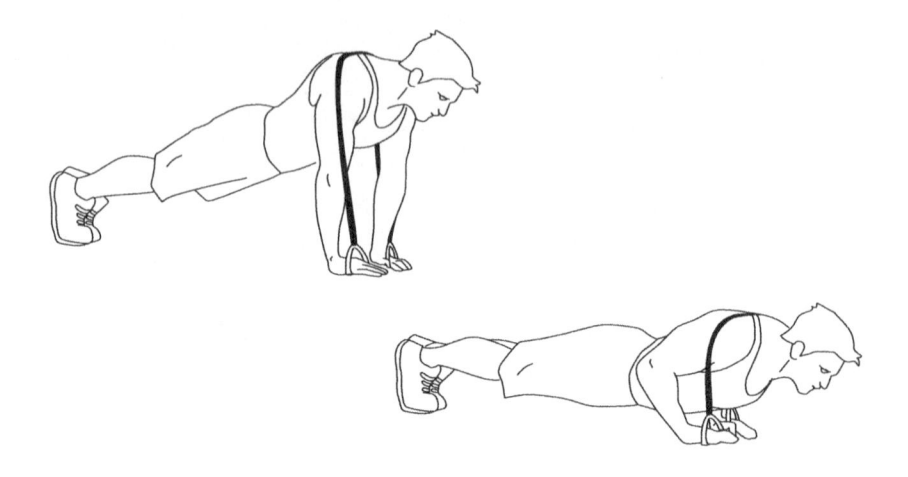

STEPS:

1 Place one end of the band on each hand between your thumb and index finger.

2 With your hands facing forward, lift the resistance band above your head and bring it down behind your back. Make sure the band is in line with your chest.

3 Get into a close grip push-up position (regular position, but with hands close together). Secure the ends of the band under your palms.

Go down slowly, extending your elbows to the side, then push back up. Repeat for your desired number of reps.

VARIATIONS:

Easier: Perform the exercise without a resistance band, only using bodyweight.

Harder: Perform the exercise with a more difficult level of resistance band.

OTHER BANDS THAT CAN BE USED:

Tube band, therapy band-similar steps.

CHAPTER 8: ARMS

BANDED CURLS-BICEPS

RESISTANCE BAND REQUIRED: Tube band

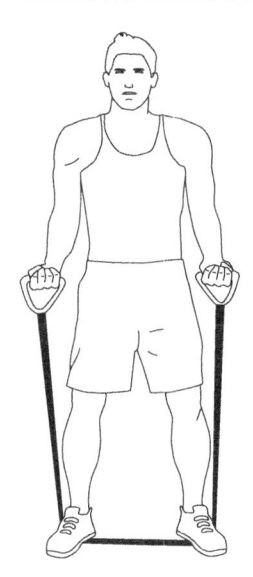

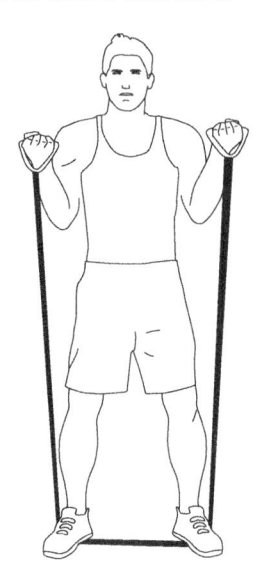

STEPS:

1 Step on the middle of the band with both feet.

2 Grab the handles so that your knuckles are facing back, at about hip height.

3 Pull the handles up to your chest. Ensure that your hands do all the pulling and your elbows stay in place. Bring back down slowly and repeat for your desired number of reps.

VARIATIONS:

Easier: Bring your feet closer together when stepping on the band to lessen resistance.

Harder: Bring your feet further apart when stepping on the band to increase resistance.

OTHER BANDS THAT CAN BE USED:

Therapy band, power resistance loop band-similar steps.

CHAPTER 8: ARMS

KNEELING SINGLE-ARM CURLS-BICEPS

RESISTANCE BAND REQUIRED: Mini loop band

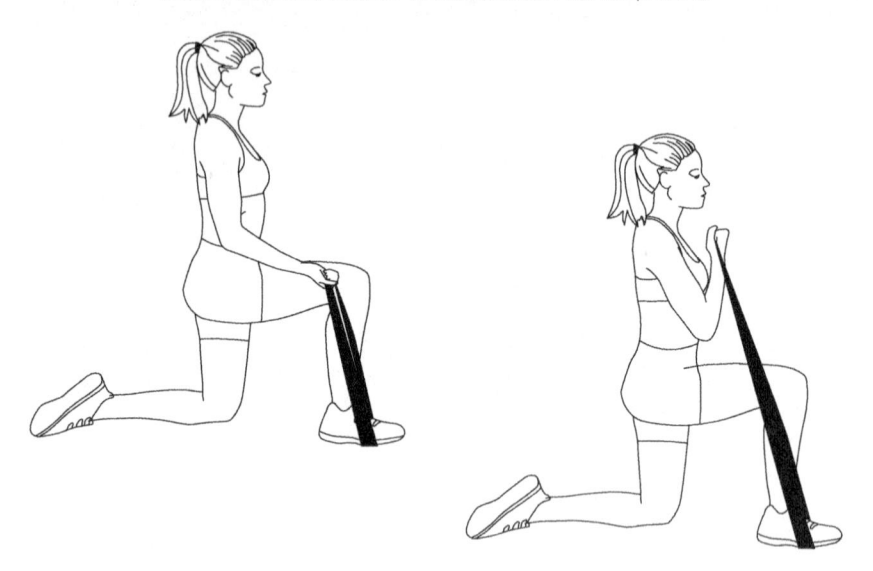

STEPS:

1 Kneel down with one leg in front and one at the back, both at about 90-degree angles.

2 Step on the bottom end of the band with your front foot. Use the hand from the same side as your foot to hold the loose end of the band, knuckles facing down, arms straight, an elbow on the knee.

3 Pull the resistance band up towards your chest. Gently bring back down and repeat for your desired number of reps. Switch sides.

VARIATIONS:

Easier: Perform the exercise using a less difficult level of resistance band.

Harder: Grab further down the resistance band. This increases resistance.

OTHER BANDS THAT CAN BE USED:

Tube band, power resistance loop band-since these bands are longer, you would need to step closer to the ends to provide adequate resistance.

CHAPTER 8: ARMS

BANDED WIDE CURLS-BICEPS

RESISTANCE BAND REQUIRED: Tube band

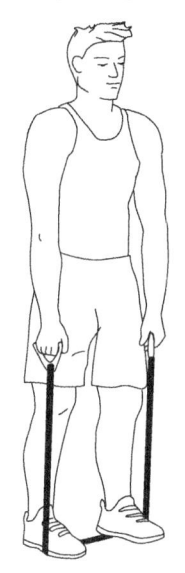

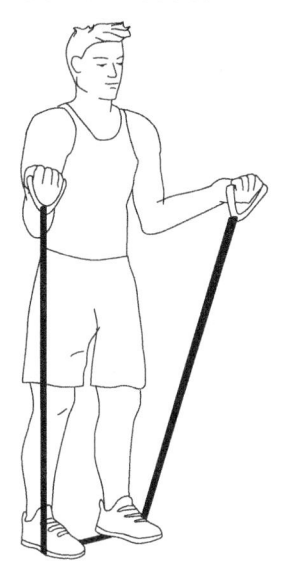

STEPS:

1 Step on the middle of the band with both feet.

2 Grab the handles and hold them out to your sides, knuckles facing outwards, arms straight.

3 Lift the handles up towards your shoulders, keeping your elbows still. Gently bring it back down. Repeat for your desired number of reps.

VARIATIONS:

Easier: Bring your feet closer together when stepping on the band to lessen resistance.

Harder: Bring your feet further apart when stepping on the band to increase resistance.

OTHER BANDS THAT CAN BE USED:

Therapy band, power resistance loop band-similar steps.

CHAPTER 8: ARMS

BANDED ALTERNATING CURLS WITH STATIC HOLD- BICEPS

RESISTANCE BAND REQUIRED: Tube band

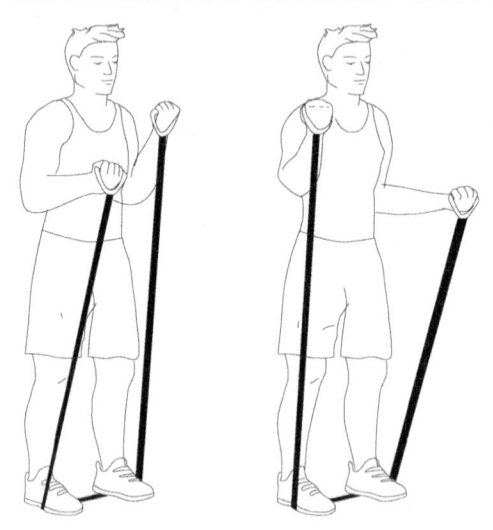

STEPS:

1 Step on the middle of the band with both feet.

2 Grab the handles so that your knuckles are facing back, hold to hip height.

3 Lift the handles up until your arms make 90-degree angles. Do curls one arm at a time, alternating with the other. When bringing your arms back down, only bring it down 90-degrees. Repeat for your desired number of reps.

VARIATIONS:

Easier-Bring your feet closer together when stepping on the band to lessen resistance.

Harder-Bring your feet further apart when stepping on the band to increase resistance.

OTHER BANDS THAT CAN BE USED:

Therapy band, power resistance loop band-similar steps.

CHAPTER 8: ARMS

BENT-OVER BANDED CURLS–BICEPS

RESISTANCE BAND REQUIRED: Tube band

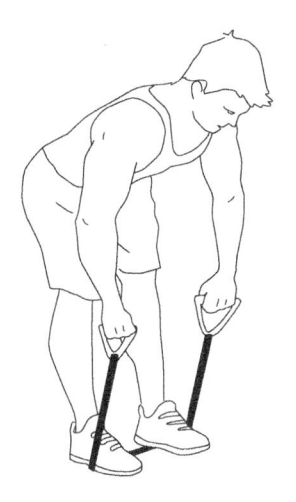

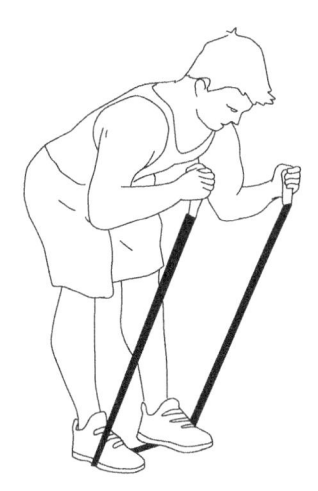

STEPS:

1 Step on the middle of the band with both feet. Grab each handle so that your knuckles are facing back, hold to hip height.

2 Bend over until your body makes a 90-degree angle. Your arms should be straight below you.

3 Pull the handles up to your face, curling your arms, ensuring that your elbows stay in place. Bring back down slowly. Repeat for your desired number of reps.

VARIATIONS:

Easier: Bring your feet closer together when stepping on the band to lessen resistance.

Harder: Bring your feet further apart when stepping on the band to increase resistance.

OTHER BANDS THAT CAN BE USED:

Power resistance loop band, therapy band–similar steps.

CHAPTER 8: ARMS

BANDED HAMMER CURLS-BICEPS

RESISTANCE BAND REQUIRED: Power resistance loop band

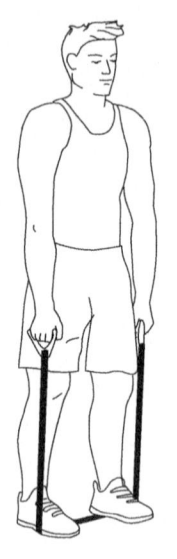

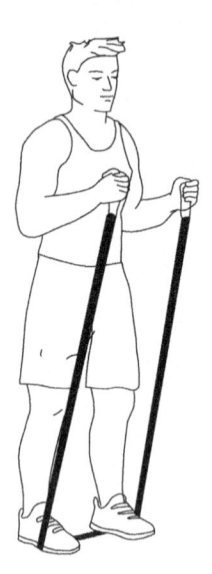

STEPS:

1 Step on the middle of the band with both feet.

2 Grab each end of the band, holding them so that your knuckles are facing out to the side, hold to about hip height with straight arms.

3 Pull the ends up to your chest. Ensure that your hands do all the pulling and your elbows stay in place. Bring back down slowly and repeat for your desired number of reps.

VARIATIONS:

Easier: Bring your feet closer together when stepping on the band to lessen resistance.

Harder: Bring your feet further apart when stepping on the band to increase resistance.

OTHER BANDS THAT CAN BE USED:

Therapy band, tube band-similar steps.

CHAPTER 8: ARMS

SEATED BANDED WRIST CURLS-FOREARMS

RESISTANCE BAND REQUIRED: Power resistance loop band

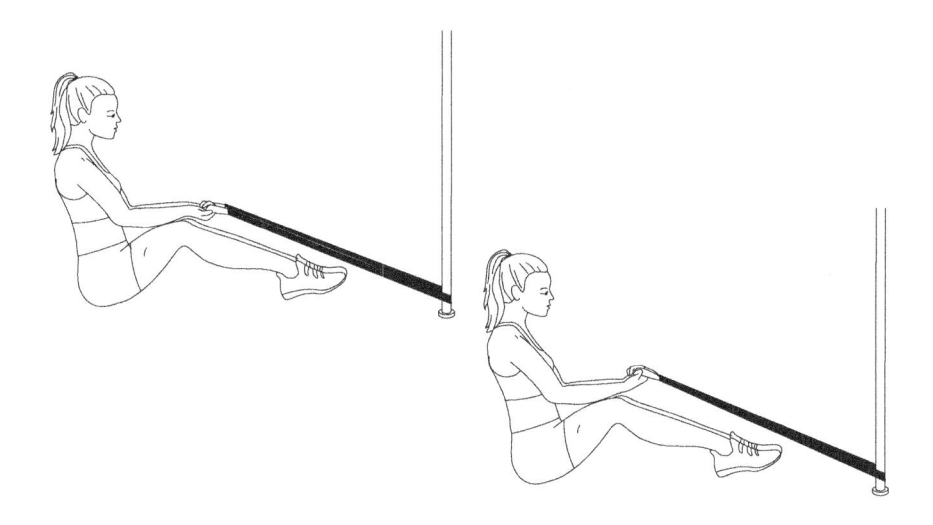

STEPS:

1 Secure the resistance band to an object that is low to the floor. Things like a table leg or pole should work well.

2 Walk the resistance band to a comfortable distance.

Sit on the floor with your knees up, thighs at an incline. Grab both handles with knuckles facing down

3 and place your arms on your thighs, with only your hands extending out.

Curl your wrists in, then out. Make sure only your wrists are doing the work. Repeat for your desired number of reps.

VARIATIONS:

Easier: Walk back closer to the object the resistance band is wrapped around on. This decreases resistance.

Harder: Walk further from the object the resistance band is wrapped around on. This increases resistance.

OTHER BANDS THAT CAN BE USED:

Tube band, mini loop band-similar steps (the mini loop band will offer a more challenging resistance).

CHAPTER 8: ARMS

SEATED BANDED PRONATED WRIST CURLS- FOREARMS

RESISTANCE BAND REQUIRED: Power resistance loop band

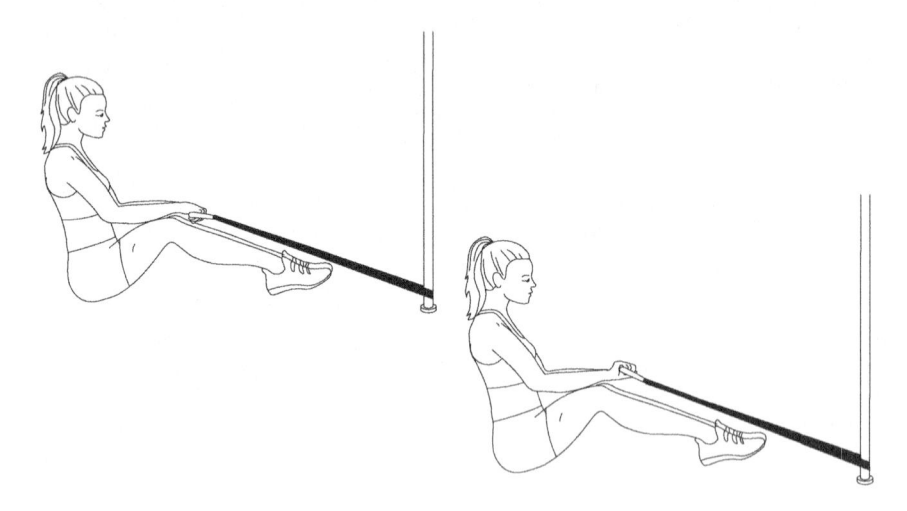

STEPS:

1 Secure the resistance band to an object that is low to the floor. Things like a table leg or pole should work well. Walk the resistance band to a comfortable distance.

2 Sit on the floor with your knees up, thighs at an incline. Grab both handles with knuckles facing up and place your arms on your thighs, with only your hands extending out.

3 Curl your wrists out, then in. Make sure only your wrists are doing the work. Repeat for your desired number of reps.

VARIATIONS:

Easier: Move back closer to the object the resistance band is wrapped around on. This decreases resistance.

Harder: Move further from the object the resistance band is wrapped around on. This increases resistance.

OTHER BANDS THAT CAN BE USED:

Tube band, mini loop band-similar steps (the mini loop band will offer a more challenging resistance).

* *Note that the change in how you hold the resistance band enables different parts of the forearms to be targeted, making this exercise different from normal seated banded wrist curls.*

CHAPTER 8: ARMS

STANDING BANDED WRIST CURLS-FOREARMS

RESISTANCE BAND REQUIRED: Tube band

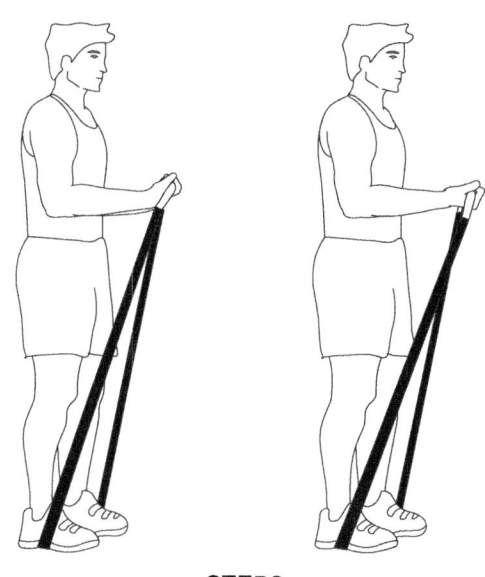

STEPS:

1 Step on the middle of the band with both feet.	**2** Grab the handles so that your knuckles are facing back, at about hip height.	**3** Lift the handles up until your arms make 90-degree angles. Curl your wrists in, then back out. Repeat for your desired number of reps.

VARIATIONS:

Easier: Bring your feet closer together when stepping on the band to lessen resistance.

Harder: Bring your feet further apart when stepping on the band to increase resistance.

OTHER BANDS THAT CAN BE USED:

Power resistance loop band-similar steps.

CHAPTER 8: ARMS

STANDING BANDED PRONATED WRIST CURLS- FOREARMS

RESISTANCE BAND REQUIRED: Tube band

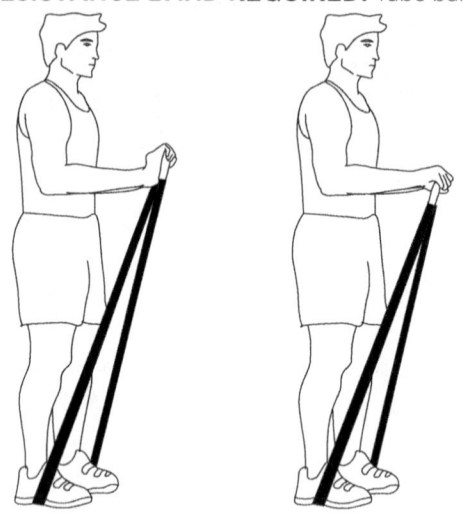

STEPS:

1 Step on the middle of the band with both feet.

2 Grab both handles so that your knuckles are facing up, at about hip height.

3 Lift the handles up until your arms make 90-degree angles. Curl your wrists in, then back out. Repeat for your desired number of reps.

VARIATIONS:

Easier: Bring your feet closer together when stepping on the band to lessen resistance.

Harder: Bring your feet further apart when stepping on the band to increase resistance.

OTHER BANDS THAT CAN BE USED:

Power resistance loop band-similar steps.

CHAPTER 8: ARMS

STANDING WRIST CIRCLES-FOREARMS

RESISTANCE BAND REQUIRED: Tube band

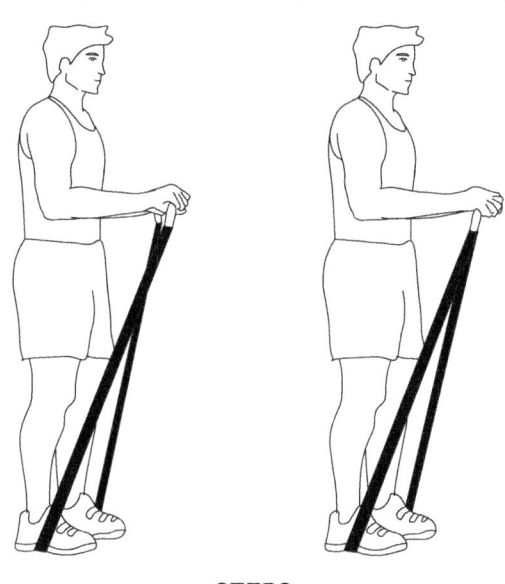

STEPS:

1 Tie the middle of the resistance band around any stable object that allows the band to be about chest level. Examples of this are a pole, or door handles.

2 With your front facing the band, grab both handles so that your knuckles are facing up. Walk the band back to a comfortable distance.

3 With straight arms, rotate both your wrists around in circles. One full rotation is one rep. Repeat for your desired number of reps.

VARIATIONS:

Easier: Walk back closer to the object the resistance band is wrapped around on. This decreases resistance.

Harder: Walk further from the object the resistance band is wrapped around on. This increases resistance.

OTHER BANDS THAT CAN BE USED:

Power resistance loop band-Similar steps.

CHAPTER 9:
LEGS

BANDED GLUTE BRIDGES
RESISTANCE BAND REQUIRED: Mini loop band

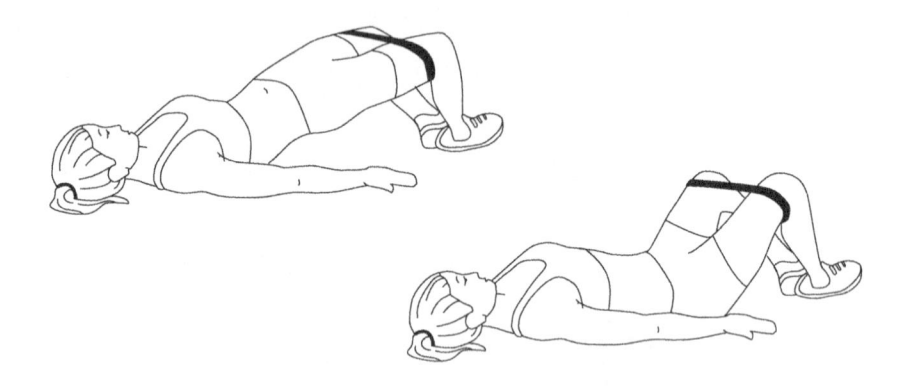

STEPS:

1 Wrap the resistance band around both legs, slightly above the knees.

2 Lie down face up on a flat surface, with your legs bent.

3 Lift your hips up as high as you can, or until your knees, chest and hips are aligned. Bring back down, then repeat for your desired number of reps.

VARIATIONS:
Easier: Execute the exercise without a resistance band, only using bodyweight.

Harder: Spread your legs further apart. This increases resistance.

OTHER BANDS THAT CAN BE USED:
Therapy band, power resistance loop band-Similar steps, but these bands need to be wrapped around multiple times as they are longer than the mini loop band.

CHAPTER 9: LEGS

BANDED SQUATS

RESISTANCE BAND REQUIRED: Power resistance loop band

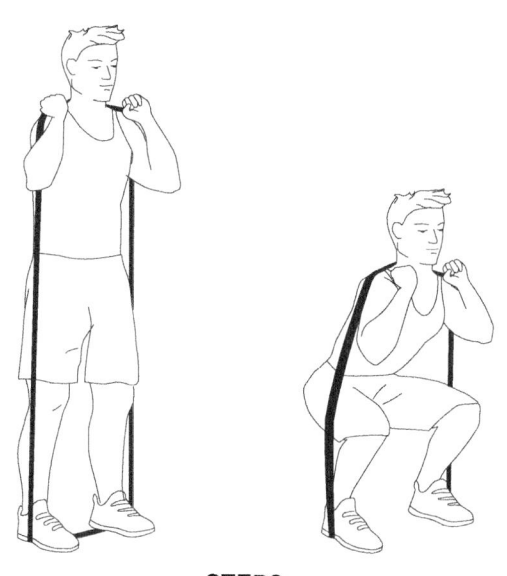

STEPS:

1. Step on the middle of the band with both feet.
2. Grab each end of the band and hold them to be above your shoulders.
3. Squat straight down, chest straight, knees out. Go back up to the starting position and repeat for your desired number of reps.

VARIATIONS:

Easier: Bring your feet closer together when stepping on the band to lessen resistance.

Harder: Bring your feet further apart when stepping on the band to increase resistance.

OTHER BANDS THAT CAN BE USED:

Therapy band, tube band-similar steps.

CHAPTER 9: LEGS

SQUAT AND JUMP

RESISTANCE BAND REQUIRED: Mini loop band

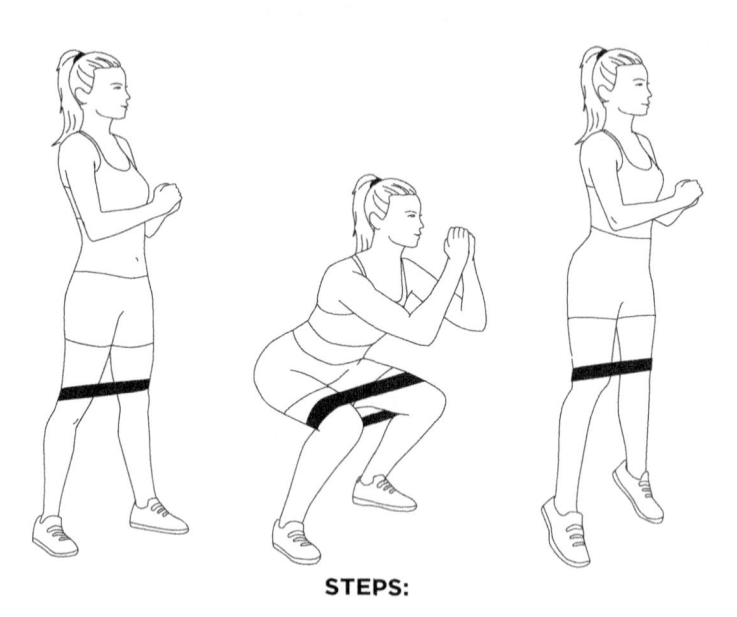

STEPS:

1 Wrap the resistance band around both legs, slightly above the knees.

2 Stand with your feet shoulder-width apart.

3 Squat down, then jump up while bringing both of your legs out to the side; perform a wide squat, then jump up, bringing your legs back shoulder-width apart. Jump back and forth doing a normal and a wide squat. Repeat for your desired number of reps.

VARIATIONS:

Easier: Perform the exercise without a resistance band, only using bodyweight.

Harder: Bring the resistance band closer to your ankles to make it more difficult.

OTHER BANDS THAT CAN BE USED:

Therapy band, power resistance loop band-Similar steps, but these bands need to be wrapped around multiple times as they are longer than the mini loop band.

CHAPTER 9: LEGS

LATERAL SIDE STEPS

RESISTANCE BAND REQUIRED: Mini loop band

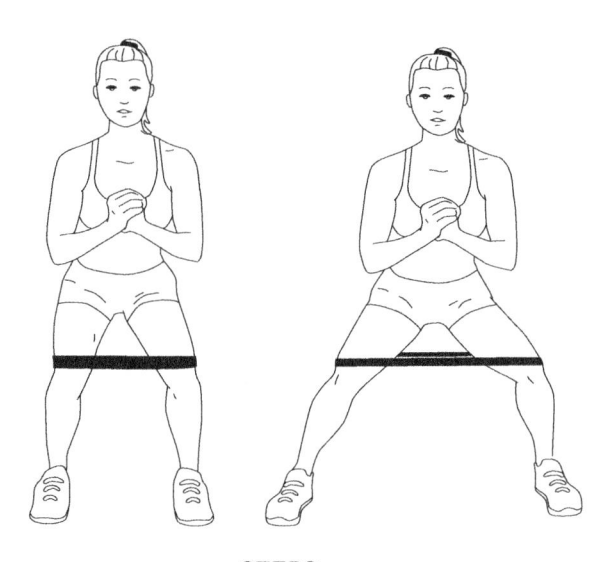

STEPS:

1 Wrap the resistance band around both legs, slightly above the knees.

2 Stand with your feet shoulder-width apart, leaning slightly forward.

3 With one foot, step out to the side, then follow with the other foot so that your feet are shoulder-width apart again. Repeat for your desired number of reps.

VARIATIONS:

Easier: Bring the resistance band close to your hips to make it easier

Harder: Bring the resistance band closer to your ankles to make it more difficult.

OTHER BANDS THAT CAN BE USED:

Therapy band, power resistance loop band-Similar steps, but these bands need to be wrapped around multiple times as they are longer than the mini loop band.

CHAPTER 9: LEGS

BANDED KICKBACKS
RESISTANCE BAND REQUIRED: Mini loop band

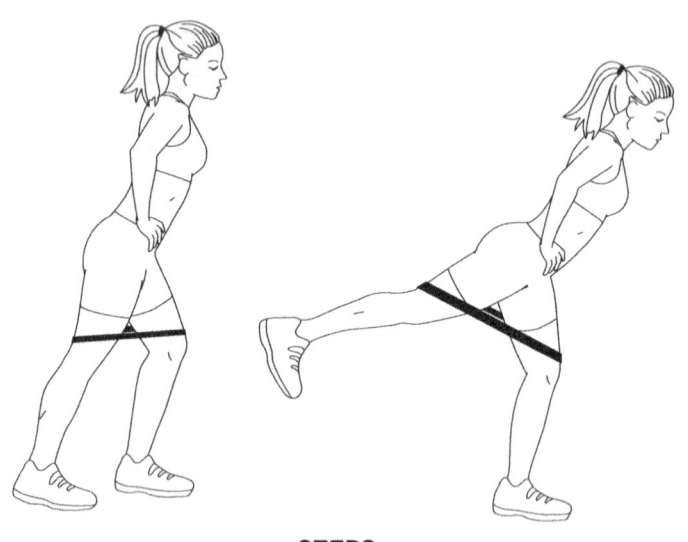

STEPS:

1 Wrap the resistance band around both legs, slightly above the knees.

2 Stand with your feet close together, leaning slightly forward.

3 Kick one leg backward as far as you can, as straight as possible. Bring back down slowly and kick back with the other leg. Alternate for your desired number of reps.

VARIATIONS:
Easier: Bring the resistance band close to your hips to make it easier

Harder: Bring the resistance band closer to your ankles to make it more difficult.

OTHER BANDS THAT CAN BE USED:

Therapy band, power resistance loop band-Similar steps, but these bands need to be wrapped around multiple times as they are longer than the mini loop band.

Tube band-needs to be tied around a low object, with the handles being attached to one foot.

CHAPTER 9: LEGS

BANDED SIDE LEG LIFTS

RESISTANCE BAND REQUIRED: Mini loop band

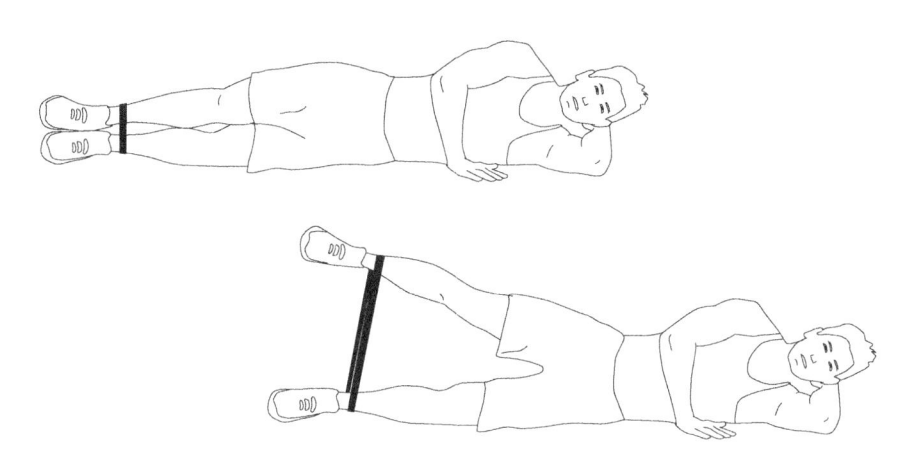

STEPS:

1. Wrap the resistance band around both legs, near the ankles.
2. Stand with your feet shoulder-width apart.
3. Bring one leg out to the side as far as you can, then gently bring it back down. Repeat for your desired number of reps. Switch legs.

VARIATIONS:

Easier: Bring the resistance band closer to your knees to make it easier.

Harder: Before bringing your leg back down, hold it out for about 3 seconds.

OTHER BANDS THAT CAN BE USED:

Therapy band, power resistance loop band-Similar steps, but these bands need to be wrapped around multiple times as they are longer than the mini loop band.

CHAPTER 9: LEGS

MID-BRIDGE IN & OUTS

RESISTANCE BAND REQUIRED: Mini loop band

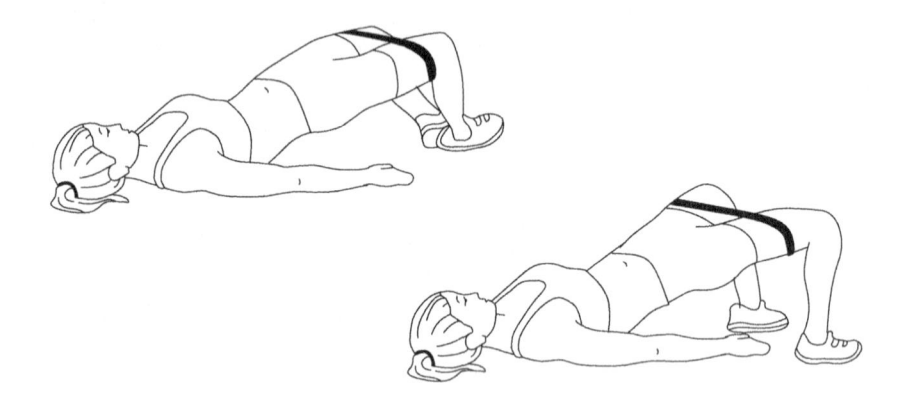

STEPS:

1 Wrap the resistance band around both legs, slightly above the knees.

2 Lie down face up on a flat surface, with your legs bent. Lift your hips up as high as you can, doing a glute bridge.

3 Bring your knees out to the side, then back in. Repeat for your desired number of reps.

VARIATIONS:

Easier: Execute the exercise without a resistance band, only using bodyweight.

Harder: Wrap the mini loop band around your legs twice over to greatly increase resistance.

OTHER BANDS THAT CAN BE USED:

Therapy band, power resistance loop band-Similar steps, but these bands need to be wrapped around multiple times as they are longer than the mini loop band.

CHAPTER 9: LEGS

BANDED BACK LUNGES

RESISTANCE BAND REQUIRED: Power resistance loop band

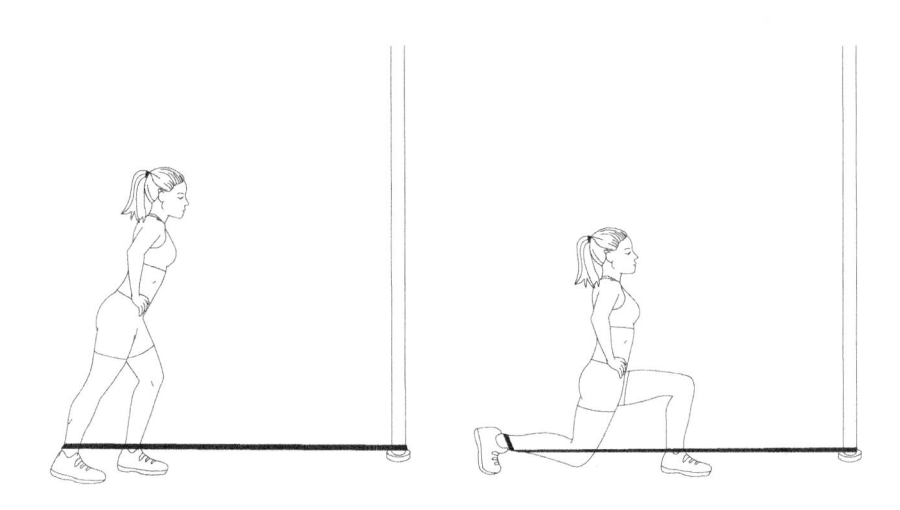

STEPS:

1. Secure the resistance band to an object that is low to the floor. Things like a table leg or pole should work well.

2. While facing the resistance band, attach the loose end to one leg near the ankles. Walk the band out to a comfortable distance.

3. Step back with the leg the band is attached to until both legs form 90-degree angles. Bring back to the starting position and repeat for your desired number of reps. Switch legs.

VARIATIONS:

Easier: Walk back closer to the object the resistance band is wrapped around on. This decreases resistance.

Harder: Walk further from the object the resistance band is wrapped around on. This increases resistance.

OTHER BANDS THAT CAN BE USED:

Tube band-similar steps.

Therapy band-similar steps but has to be tied around both the object and your ankles.

CHAPTER 9: LEGS

TABLETOP SIDE LEG RAISES

RESISTANCE BAND REQUIRED: Mini loop band

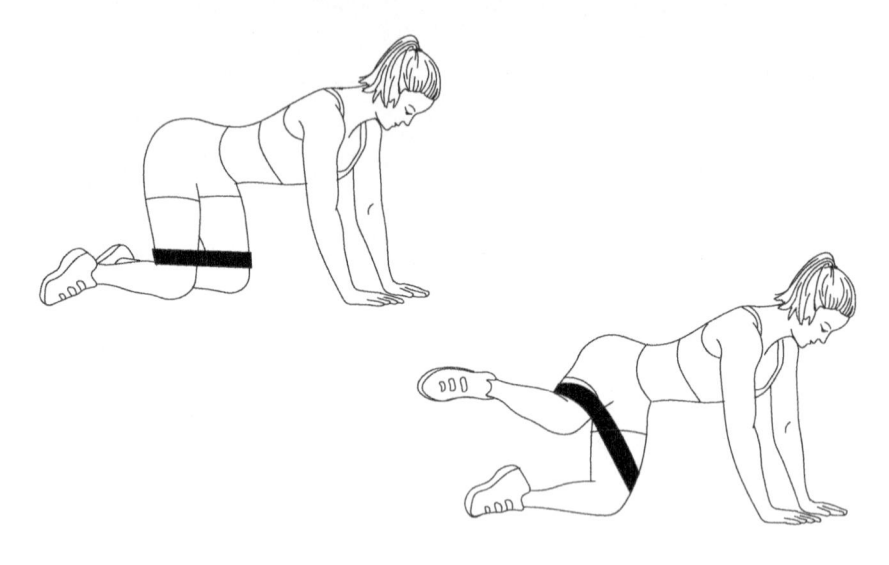

STEPS:

1 Wrap the resistance band around both legs, slightly above the knees.

2 Place yourself on the floor, face down, on all fours.

3 Bring one leg out to the side as far as you can, keeping your hips in place. Bring gently back down and repeat for your desired number of reps. Switch legs.

VARIATIONS:

Easier-perform the exercise without a resistance band, only using bodyweight.

Harder-before bringing your leg back down, hold it out for about 3 seconds.

OTHER BANDS THAT CAN BE USED:

Therapy band, power resistance loop band-Similar steps, but these bands need to be wrapped around multiple times as they are longer than the mini loop band.

CHAPTER 9: LEGS

BANDED TABLETOP KICKBACKS

RESISTANCE BAND REQUIRED: Mini loop band

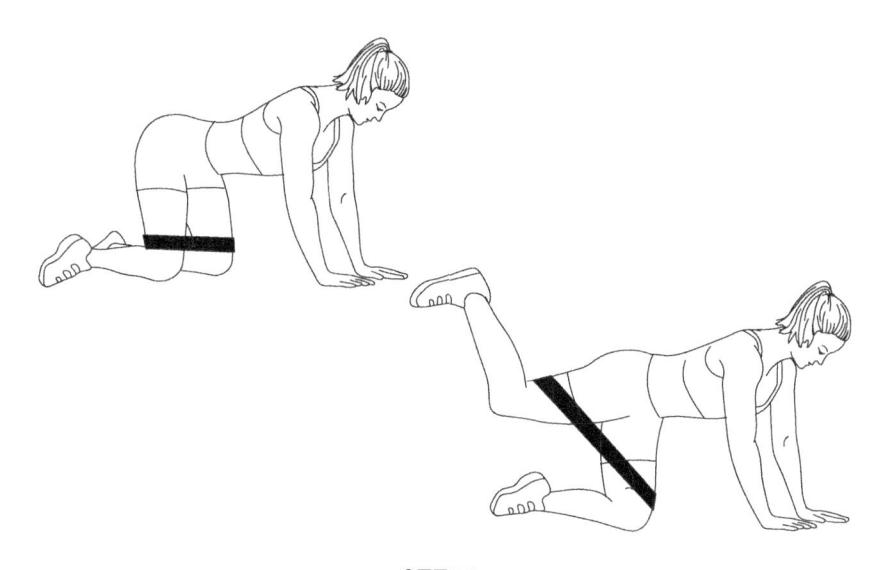

STEPS:

1. Wrap the resistance band around both legs, slightly above the knees.
2. Place yourself on the floor, face down, on all fours.
3. Kick one leg back, then up as far as you can. Gently bring back down and repeat for your desired number of reps. Switch legs.

VARIATIONS:

Easier: Perform the exercise with an easier level of a resistance band or no resistance band at all.

Harder: Wrap the mini loop band around your legs twice over to greatly increase resistance.

OTHER BANDS THAT CAN BE USED:

Therapy band, power resistance loop band-Similar steps, but these bands need to be wrapped around multiple times as they are longer than the mini loop band.

CHAPTER 9: LEGS

BANDED CALF RAISES

RESISTANCE BAND REQUIRED: Power resistance loop band

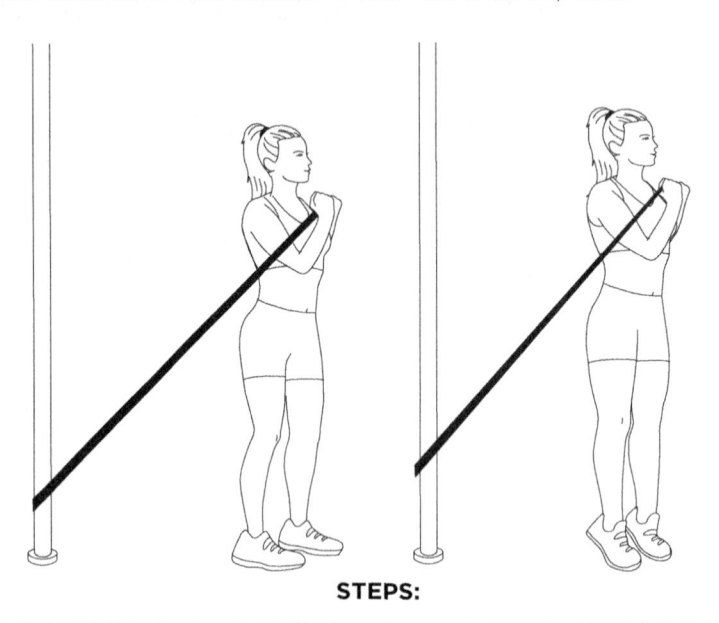

STEPS:

1 Secure the resistance band to an object that is low to the floor. Things like a table leg or pole should work well.

2 With your back towards the resistance band, grab the loose end with both hands. Lift the band up behind you to shoulder height, spreading your hands apart so that one hand is on each shoulder.

3 Slowly stand up to your tippy toes, hold for a second, then slowly bring back down. Repeat for your desired number of reps.

VARIATIONS:

Easier: Move back closer to the object the resistance band is wrapped around on. This decreases resistance.

Harder: Move further from the object the resistance band is wrapped around on. This increases resistance.

OTHER BANDS THAT CAN BE USED:

Tube band, therapy band-similar steps, but the band needs to be secured in the middle instead of the end. This is so both handles are free.

CHAPTER 9: LEGS

BANDED SQUAT CALF RAISES

RESISTANCE BAND REQUIRED: Mini loop band

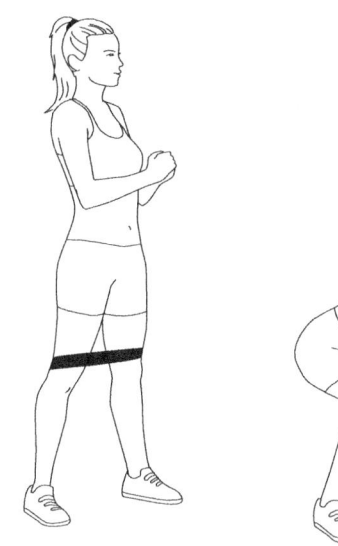

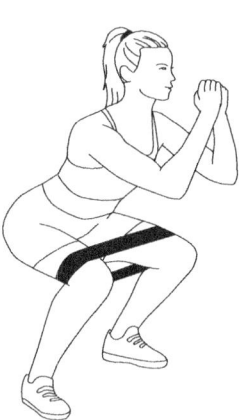

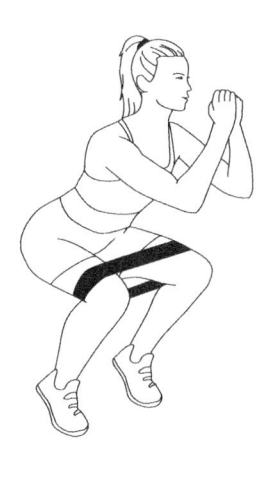

STEPS:

1 Wrap the resistance band around both legs, slightly above the knees.

2 Stand with your feet shoulder-width apart.

Squat down, keeping your back straight, knees pointed out. When you get to the bottom, stand on your toes.

3 Hold for a second, then slowly bring back down and rise back up. Repeat for your desired number of reps.

VARIATIONS:

Easier: Perform the exercise without a resistance band, only using bodyweight.

Harder: Before going back down, hold the squat and/or the calf raise for longer.

OTHER BANDS THAT CAN BE USED:

Therapy band, power resistance loop band-Similar steps, but these bands need to be wrapped around multiple times as they are longer than the mini loop band.

CHAPTER 10:
CORE

BANDED RUSSIAN TWISTS

RESISTANCE BAND REQUIRED: Power resistance loop band

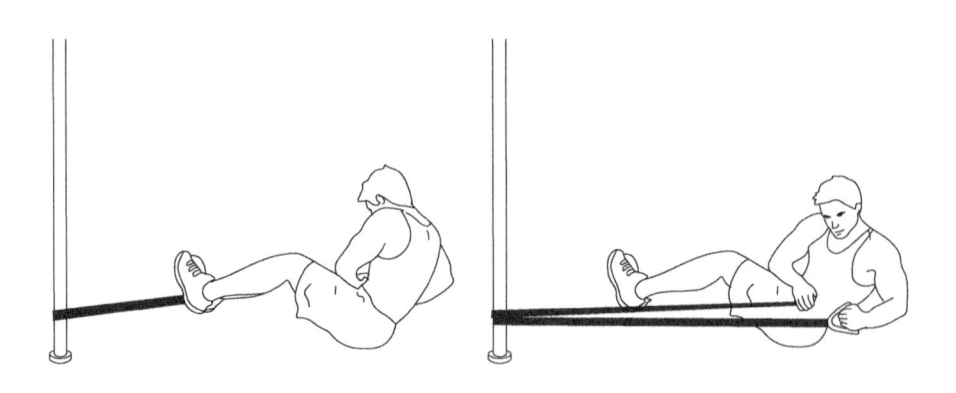

STEPS:

1 Secure the resistance band to an object that is low to the floor. Things like a table leg or pole should work well. Walk the band to a comfortable distance.

2 With your front facing the band, sit down with your legs straight in front of you. Hold the end of the resistance band with both hands.

3 Lean back slightly and lift your legs up, still keeping them straight. Then, with your core tight, twist your torso from side to side while holding the resistance band. Repeat for your desired number of reps.

VARIATIONS:

Easier: Perform the exercise without a resistance band, or move closer to the object the band is secured on.

Harder: Move further from the object the resistance band is wrapped around on. This increases resistance.

OTHER BANDS THAT CAN BE USED:

Therapy band, tube band-similar steps.

CHAPTER 10: CORE

BANDED LYING LEG RAISES

RESISTANCE BAND REQUIRED: Power resistance loop band

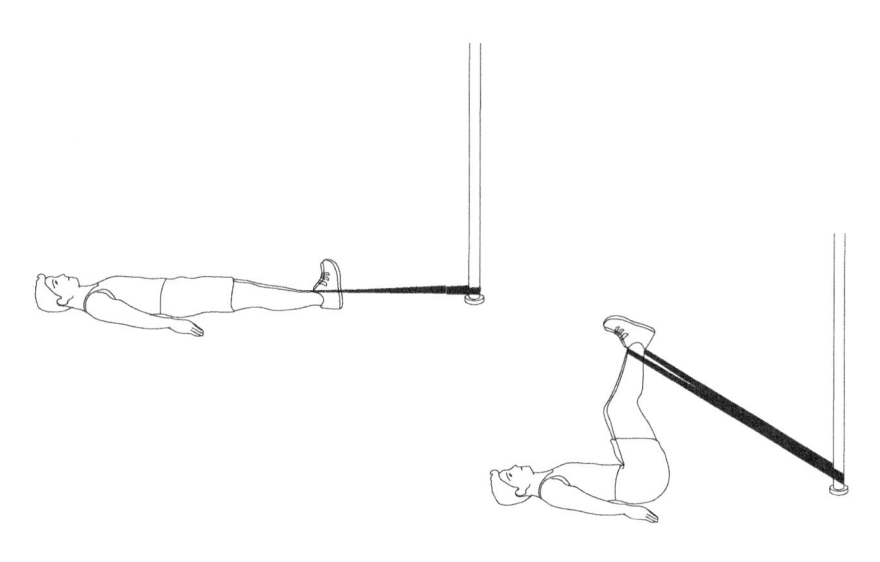

STEPS:

1 Secure the resistance band to an object that is low to the floor. Things like a table leg or pole should work well. Walk the band to a comfortable distance.

2 With your front facing the band, secure the loose end to both of your feet. Lie down on a flat surface with your feet straight out, hands flat to the side.

3 With your core tight, lift your legs up while keeping them straight, bringing the resistance band with it. Gently bring it back down, but don't touch the floor. Repeat for your desired number of reps.

VARIATIONS:

Easier-perform the exercise without a resistance band, or move closer to the object the band is secured on.

Harder-walk further from the object the resistance band is wrapped around on. This increases resistance.

OTHER BANDS THAT CAN BE USED:

Tube band, therapy band-similar steps.

CHAPTER 10: CORE

BANDED LYING KNEE TUCK INS

RESISTANCE BAND REQUIRED: Power resistance loop band

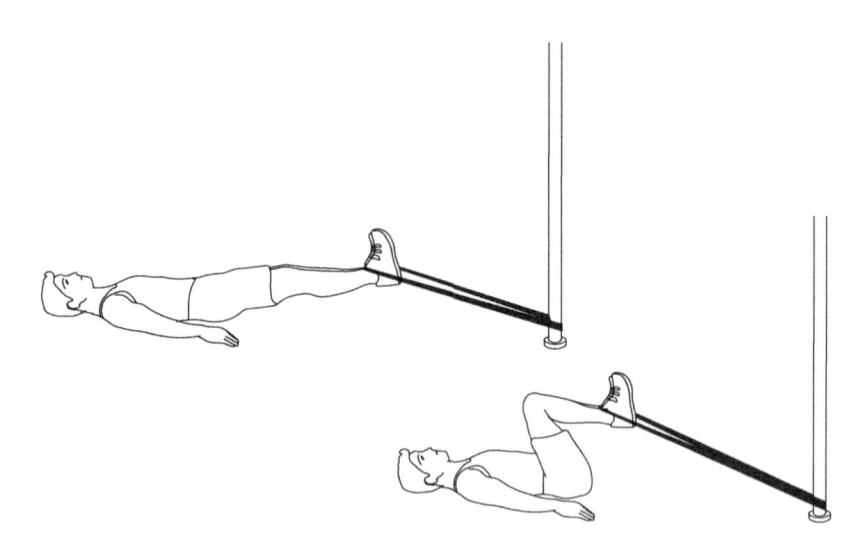

STEPS:

1. Secure the resistance band to an object that is low to the floor. Things like a table leg or pole should work well. Walk the band to a comfortable distance.

2. With your front facing the band, secure the loose end to both of your feet. Lie down on a flat surface with your feet straight out, hands flat to the side.

3. Lift your feet slightly up, then bring your knees in towards you until they form a 90-degree angle. Slowly bring back out but don't touch the floor. Repeat for your desired number of reps.

VARIATIONS:

Easier: Move back closer to the object the resistance band is wrapped around on. This decreases resistance.

Harder: Move further from the object the resistance band is wrapped around on. This increases resistance.

OTHER BANDS THAT CAN BE USED:

Tube band, therapy band-similar steps.

CHAPTER 10: CORE

BANDED BICYCLES

RESISTANCE BAND REQUIRED: Mini loop band

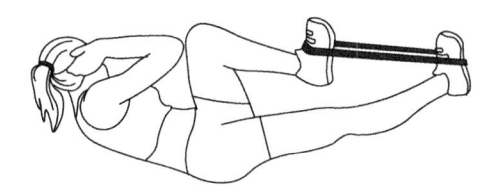

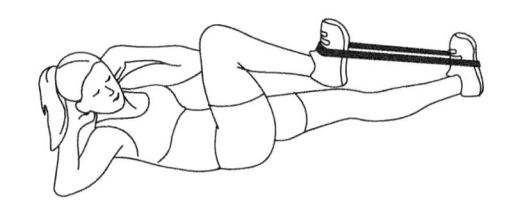

STEPS:

1 Secure the resistance band around both of your feet. Lie down on a flat surface, face up.

2 To start, lift your head up to about a 45-degree angle and put your hands behind your head, elbows facing out. Lift your legs by bringing your knees towards you.

3 Extend one leg out while bringing the other to touch your elbow (left knee to right elbow, right knee to left elbow).

Bring that leg back in a while, preparing to extend the other leg. Repeat for your desired number of reps.

VARIATIONS:

Easier: Perform the exercise without a resistance band, only using bodyweight.

Harder: Spread your feet further apart in the starting position to create more resistance.

OTHER BANDS THAT CAN BE USED:

Therapy band, power resistance loop band-Similar steps, but these bands need to be wrapped around multiple times as they are longer than the mini loop band.

CHAPTER 10: CORE

BANDED SCISSOR KICKS

RESISTANCE BAND REQUIRED: Mini loop band

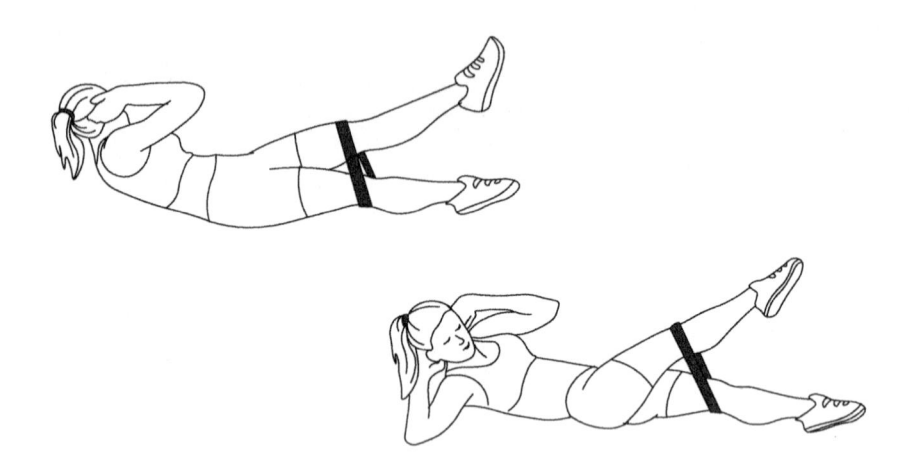

STEPS:

1 Wrap the resistance band around both legs, slightly above the knees.

2 Lie down on a flat surface, face up, hand flat to the side, legs straight.

3 With your core tight, bring one leg straight up while keeping the other down. As you bring that leg back down, bring the other leg up. Alternate for your desired number of reps.

VARIATIONS:

Easier: Perform the exercise without resistance, only using bodyweight.

Harder: Bring the resistance band closer to your ankles to make it more difficult.

OTHER BANDS THAT CAN BE USED:

Therapy band, power resistance loop band-Similar steps, but these bands need to be wrapped around multiple times as they are longer than the mini loop band.

CHAPTER 10: CORE

BANDED SIDE PLANK RAISES

RESISTANCE BAND REQUIRED: Mini loop band

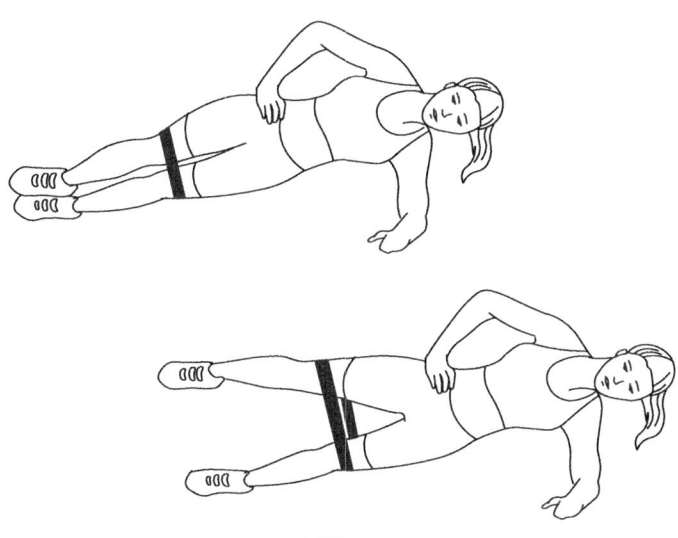

STEPS:

1 Wrap the resistance band around both legs, slightly above the knees.

2 Lie down on your side. Lift your hips up by using your arm as support. Keep your legs together, one leg above the other.

3 Lift the leg that is above up as far as you can, then gently bring it back down. Repeat for your desired number of reps. Switch sides.

VARIATIONS:

Easier: Perform the exercise without resistance, only using bodyweight.

Harder: Bring the resistance band closer to your ankles to make it more difficult.

OTHER BANDS THAT CAN BE USED:

Therapy band, power resistance loop band-Similar steps, but these bands need to be wrapped around multiple times as they are longer than the mini loop band.

CHAPTER 10: CORE

STANDING OBLIQUE TWISTS

RESISTANCE BAND REQUIRED: Power resistance loop band

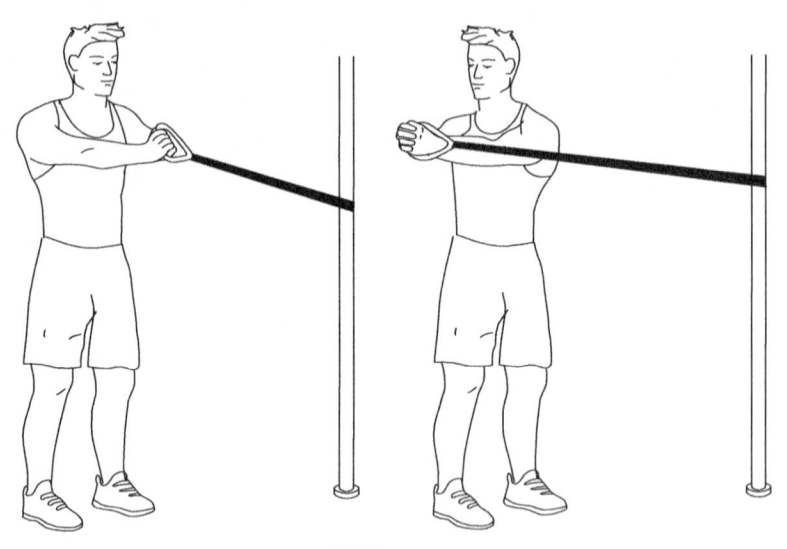

STEPS:

1 Tie the resistance band around any stable object that allows the band to be about chest level.

2 With your side facing the band, grab the loose end with both hands close together. Walk-out to a comfortable distance and hold the band out to the side where the object it's secured on with straight arms.

3 Twist your upper body, pulling the band until you have made a 180-degree turn. Bring back to the starting position and repeat for your desired number of reps.

VARIATIONS:

Easier: Move closer to the object the resistance band is wrapped around on. This decreases resistance.

Harder: Move further from the object the resistance band is wrapped around on. This increases resistance.

OTHER BANDS THAT CAN BE USED:

Therapy band, tube band-similar steps.

CHAPTER 10: CORE

KNEELING ANGLED OBLIQUE TWISTS

RESISTANCE BAND REQUIRED: Power resistance loop band

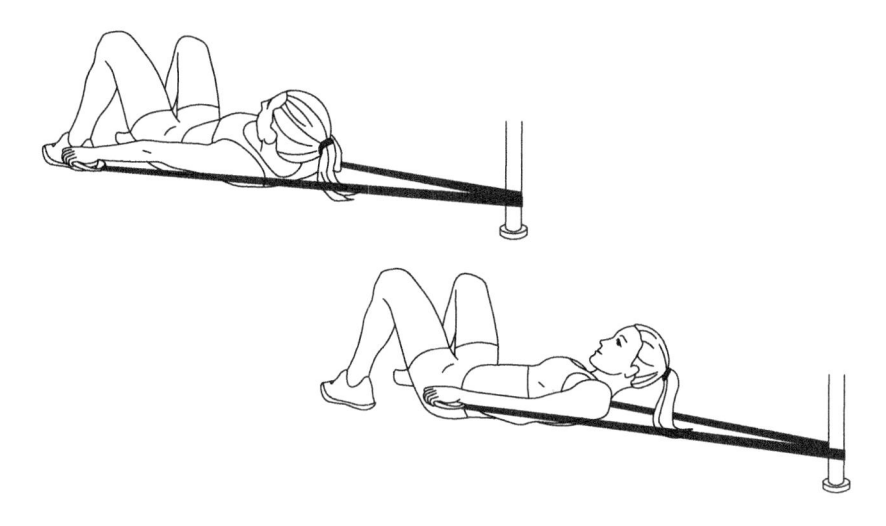

STEPS:

1 Tie the resistance band around any stable object that allows the band to be about chest level. With your side facing the band, grab the loose end with both hands close together and Walk-out to a comfortable distance.

2 Kneel down, with one leg at the front and one at the back, both at 90-degree angles. Your side should still be facing the band.

3 Hold the band out to the side where the object it's secured on with straight arms. Then, pull the band down diagonally while twisting your body until you have made a 180-degree turn. Bring the resistance band back up and repeat for your desired number of reps.

VARIATIONS:

Easier: Move closer to the object the resistance band is wrapped around on. This decreases resistance.

Harder: Move further from the object the resistance band is wrapped around on. This increases resistance.

OTHER BANDS THAT CAN BE USED:

Therapy band, tube band-similar steps.

CHAPTER 10: CORE

BANDED LYING TOE TOUCHES
RESISTANCE BAND REQUIRED: Tube band

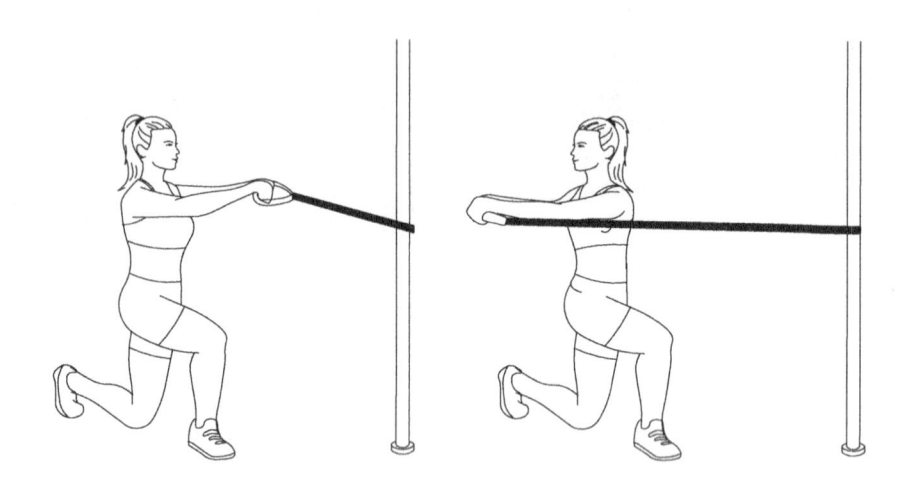

STEPS:

1 Secure the middle of the resistance band to an object that is low to the floor. Things like a table leg or pole should work well. Walk-out to a comfortable distance

2 With your back to the resistance band, lie down on the floor, legs bent. Grab the handles and hold them out to the side with straight arms. Lift your head up.

3 Move your body from side to side (but don't twist your hips), touching each heel of your foot. Alternate for your desired number of reps.

VARIATIONS:

Easier: Move closer to the object the resistance band is wrapped around on. This decreases resistance.

Harder: Move further from the object the resistance band is wrapped around on. This increases resistance.

OTHER BANDS THAT CAN BE USED:

Therapy band, power resistance loop band-similar steps.

CHAPTER 10: CORE

BANDED FLUTTER KICKS

RESISTANCE BAND REQUIRED: Power resistance loop band

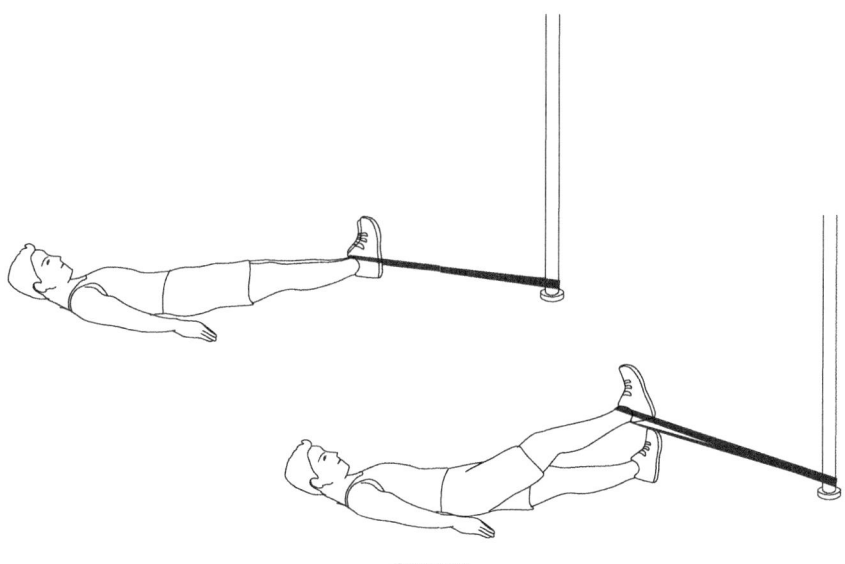

STEPS:

1. Secure the middle of the resistance band to an object that is low to the floor. Things like a table leg or pole should work well. Walk the band out to a comfortable distance.

2. With your front facing the back, lie down on the floor. Secure an end of the resistance band to a foot.

   Lift your head and legs up slightly, with your hands to the side.

3. With a tight core and straight legs, lift one leg up as high as you can, then gently bring it back down. Do the same for the other leg. Alternate for your desired number of reps.

VARIATIONS:

Easier: Perform the exercise without a resistance band, only using bodyweight. You can also move closer to the object the band is wrapped around on.

Harder: Move further from the object the resistance band is wrapped around on. This increases resistance.

OTHER BANDS THAT CAN BE USED:

Tube band-similar steps.

Therapy band-similar steps, but ends need to be tied around your feet.

CHAPTER 10: CORE

BANDED BOAT HOLD

RESISTANCE BAND REQUIRED: Therapy band

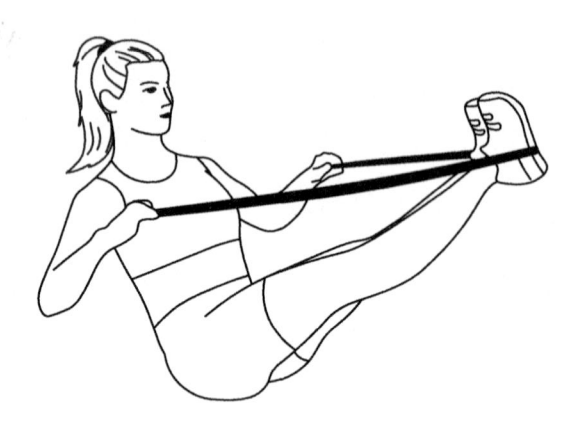

STEPS:

1 Sit down on a flat surface with your legs out and body at a 90-degree angle to your legs.

2 Secure the resistance band around both of your feet. Grab both ends and hold them out front with straight arms.

3 Lift straight legs up and lean back until your body makes about a 45-degree angle. The only thing in contact with the ground should be your butt. Pull the ends of the band towards your chest. Hold the pose for as long as you can.

VARIATIONS:

Easier: Perform the exercise without a resistance band, only using bodyweight. Just keep your hands straight out, elevated at your sides.

Harder: Grab the resistance band, so your hands are closer to the middle (not the ends). This increases tension in the core.

OTHER BANDS THAT CAN BE USED:

Power resistance loop band, tube band-Similar steps.

ALL IN ALL...

Staying fit is not easy, yes, but it's also extremely rewarding. Not only does it provide countless health benefits, but it also makes us feel accomplished and happier with our bodies. Remember, the most important thing to remember in your fitness journey is consistency! It's okay to miss a day once in a while, but being consistent maximizes gains and even trains the mind to be more motivated and learn to like hard work.

Like how going to school doesn't automatically get you a job, being knowledgeable about exercise will not get you your dream body. Remember that it is only **YOU** that'll be responsible for meeting your goals. So what are you waiting for? Plan your next workout now using these great resistance band exercises that will set you up to be well on your way into your fitness journey!

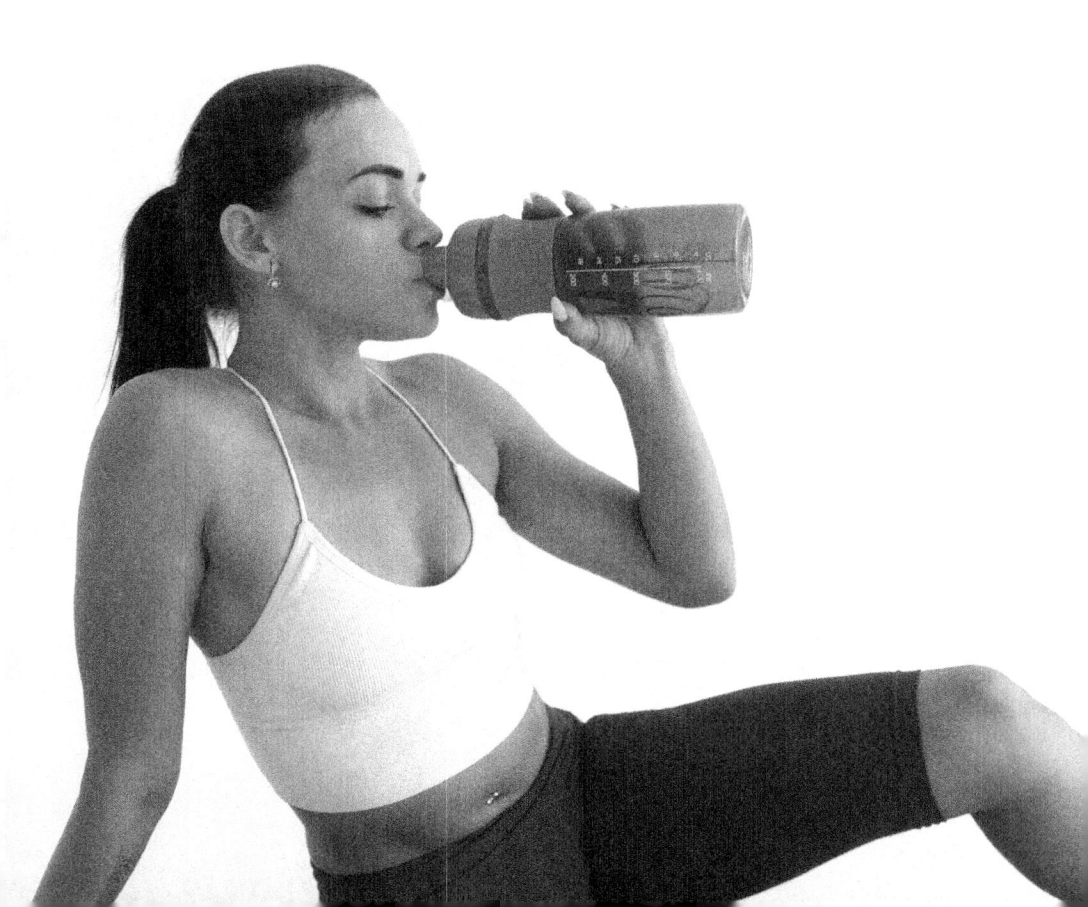

REFERENCES

5 MIN WARM UP | FULL BODY WARMUP FOR AT HOME WORKOUTS | TIFFxDAN. (2021, March 9). Www.youtube.com. https://www.youtube.com/watch?v=_6-k5-w1bZw

5 Mini Band Arm Exercises You Can Do Anywhere • The Live Fit Girls. (2019, July 1). The Live Fit Girls. https://thelivefitgirls.com/mini-band-arm-exercises/

5 Quick Resistance-Band Arm Workouts You Can Do at Home. (2018). 5 Quick Resistance-Band Arm Workouts You Can Do at Home. Byrdie. https://www.byrdie.com/resistance-band-arm-exercises

8 Back Exercises for Resistance Bands -NO ATTACHING. (2021, February 6). Www.youtube.com. https://www.youtube.com/watch?v=IP4wM2JpDdQ

11 Resistance Band Chest Exercises -NO ATTACHING. (2021, February 2). Fitgent. https://www.youtube.com/watch?v=UydUK8KLqt8

Anwar, O. (2020, August 27). 11 Resistance Band Exercises for Legs to Strengthen and Tone. Lifehack. https://www.lifehack.org/881337/resistance-band-exercises-for-legs

Benefits of resistance band training. (2020, May 1). Crunch Fitness. https://www.crunch.com.au/blog/uncategorized/benefits-of-resistance-band-training/

Bomgren, L. (2020, August). 30-Minute Resistance Band Leg Workout for Women | Legs, Glutes + Thighs. Www.youtube.com. https://www.youtube.com/watch?v=dbgP-jKARvk

Brinsley, J. (2019, January 16). 22 benefits of resistance training with an Exercise Physiologist. Exercise Right. https://exerciseright.com.au/benefits-of-resistance-training-exercise-physiologist/

Chertoff, J. (2020, July 30). Progressive Overload: What It Is, Examples, and Tips. Healthline. https://www.healthline.com/health/progressive-overload#benefits

Cronkleton, E. (2020, December 1). 6 Shoulder Exercises Using Resistance Bands. Healthline. https://www.healthline.com/health/shoulder-band-exercise#resistance-band-benefits

Determination of Resistance Training Frequency. (2017, May 1). Www.nsca.com. https://www.nsca.com/education/articles/kinetic-select/determination-of-resistance-training-frequency/#:~:text=The%20recommendation%20for%20the%20novice

Dewar, M. (n.d.). 17 Resistance Band Ab Exercise For A Strong Core – Fitbod. Retrieved July 13, 2021, from https://fitbod.me/blog/resistance-band-ab-exercises/

Edwards, T. (2021, May 6). fitness. Healthline. https://www.healthline.com/health/fitness/resistance-band-chest-workout#3-Moves-to-Strengthen-Glutes-Using-Resistance-Bands

FOREARM WORKOUT with Resistance Bands. (2010, May 27). Www.youtube.com. https://www.youtube.com/watch?v=xyHLejrielo

Galic, B. (2020, June 25). The Only 5 Resistance Band Exercises You Need for Toned Calves. Livestrong.com. https://www.livestrong.com/article/103743-resistance-band-calf-exercises/

Gear, V. (n.d.). The 9 Best Resistance Band Tricep Exercises. Victorem Gear. Retrieved

REFERENCES

July 11, 2021, from https://victoremgear.com/blogs/resistance-training/resistance-band-tricep-exercises

Goulet, C. (2019, July 15). Progressive Overload: The Concept You Must Know To Grow! Bodybuilding.com; Bodybuilding.com. https://www.bodybuilding.com/content/progressive-overload-the-concept-you-must-know-to-grow.html

Hannah. (2013, March 12). Breaking the Code of Resistance Band Colors. Medical Supplies | Home Medical Equipment | Discount Medical Supply Store. https://blog.allegromedical.com/breaking-the-code-of-resistance-band-colors-2286.html

Heria, C. (2020, November 23). Super Effective Shoulder Workout Using Only Resistance Bands. Www.youtube.com. https://www.youtube.com/watch?v=FRuiQ36x-Ik

Lefkowith, C. (2020, February 1). 17 Resistance Band Core Exercises. Www.youtube.com. https://www.youtube.com/watch?v=gcXhImYKQ_c

mainpath. (2016, December 15). Tri-City Medical Center. Tri-City Medical Center. https://www.tricitymed.org/2016/12/warming-cooling-important/

McCall, P. (2015, March 5). Fitness Terminology | 10 Popular Fitness Terms Defined. Www.acefitness.org. https://www.acefitness.org/education-and-resources/lifestyle/blog/5325/fitness-terminology-10-popular-fitness-terms-defined/

McMillan, L. (2021, April 27). Simply the Chest: The Best Resistance Band Chest Workouts. Greatist. https://greatist.com/fitness/resistance-band-chest-workout#exercises

Mike Rosa. (2020a). Resistance Band Tricep Workout At Home to Get Ripped! In YouTube. https://www.youtube.com/watch?v=EjjRIQrFCCU

Morgan, R. (2020, January 29). Resistance Band Romanian Deadlift (RDL) | Exercises to do at home | Travel Workouts. https://www.youtube.com/watch?v=2DswHFace6c

Paige Waehner. (2019). Considering How Often You Should Workout When Starting An Exercise. Verywell Fit. https://www.verywellfit.com/exercise-frequency-recommendation-1231215

Penn State Extension. (2019, August 31). Warm-up and Cool-down. Penn State Extension. https://extension.psu.edu/warm-up-and-cool-down

Quinn, E. (2003, November 24). Should You Warm up Before Exercise? Verywell Fit; Verywellfit. https://www.verywellfit.com/how-to-warm-up-before-exercise-3119266

Resistance training – health benefits. (2012). Vic.gov.au. https://www.betterhealth.vic.gov.au/health/healthyliving/resistance-training-health-benefits

Rogers, P. (2020, November 2). Pros and Cons of Split System Training. Verywell Fit. https://www.verywellfit.com/split-system-training-purpose-and-routines-3498381#:~:text=Split%20system%20training%20is%20a

Rosa, M. (2017a, July 25). Intense 5 Minute Resistance Band Shoulder Workout. Www.youtube.com. https://www.youtube.com/watch?v=AbfPO41tk68

Rosa, M. (2017b, August 29). Intense 5 Minute Resistance Band Chest Workout. Www.

REFERENCES

youtube.com. https://www.youtube.com/watch?v=sMP2F0OXRYI

Rosa, M. (2020b, September 23). Resistance Band Back Workout At Home to Get Ripped! Www.youtube.com. https://www.youtube.com/watch?v=-j44AZXcnX8

Rosa, M. (2020c, October 1). Resistance Band Leg Workout At Home to Get Ripped! Www.youtube.com. https://www.youtube.com/watch?v=u9g8rh2flrU

Rosa, M. (2020d, October 9). Resistance Band Shoulder Workout At Home to Get Ripped! Www.youtube.com. https://www.youtube.com/watch?v=ZdsGGqXn8W0

SET, S. F. (2019, April 9). 5 Types of Resistance Bands & Which Resistance Bands are the Best? SET for SET. https://www.setforset.com/blogs/news/5-types-of-resistance-bands-which-is-best-to-buy

Sollon, M. (2015, February 3). How Do You Determine Your Fitness Level? Total Gym Pulse. https://totalgymdirect.com/total-gym-blog/how-to-determine-your-fitness-level

Staff, E. (2018, August 22). 42 Gym Slang Terms: The Cheat Sheet to Gym Lingo. The Fitness Tribe. https://thefitnesstribe.com/gym-slang-terms/

Tara Hall. (n.d.). Top 8 Resistance Band Shoulder Exercises | Mirafit. Mirafit.co.uk. Retrieved July 10, 2021, from https://mirafit.co.uk/blog/best-shoulder-exercises-using-resistance-bands/

The Definitive Guide to Resistance Bands and Workout Bands. (n.d.). WODFitters. https://www.wodfitters.com/pages/the-definitive-guide-to-resistance-bands-and-workout-bands

Theifels, J. (2017, April 21). How To Breathe While Working Out, Exercising. AARP. https://www.aarp.org/health/healthy-living/info-2017/breathe-exercise-workout.html

Printed in Great Britain
by Amazon